THE
NEW THYROID
HANDBOOK

A guide for frustrated thyroid patients
and medical professionals

JEFFERY WHELCHEL, MD

CONTENTS

INTRODUCTION

DO YOU THINK YOU HAVE A THYROID ISSUE? YOU ARE PROBABLY RIGHT!

Jennifer is a 47-year-old long-time patient of mine who came to see me for an annual checkup. After catching up for a bit, the topic of conversation turned to her overall health. "I guess I'm doing okay," she told me. "I certainly don't feel as good as I used to. I'm tired and stressed, just like everyone else I know. I keep gaining a little bit of weight every year even though I'm eating less and less. I exercise sometimes, but most days, I'm just too tired to make myself do it. I have always wondered if I had a thyroid or hormone problem, but my lab work always looks good. But I'm okay. I guess this all just comes with getting older."

Does her story sound familiar? Could we be describing you or someone in your family? Would it make a difference if she were 27, or 37, or 57, or 67?

I hear similar stories constantly in my practice from people in their early 20s to their late 80s.

In the first few years of my medical practice, these kinds of stories both broke my heart and gave me immense frustration. The physical exam typically looked fine. The basic labs that I ordered would inevitably be in the normal ranges.

For a medical provider, there is nothing worse than not knowing what to do to help your patient.

Most patients won't accept leaving a doctor's visit where they have paid a substantial amount of money without getting some kind of treatment plan.

We are expected to do something, ANYTHING, to help. If not, the patient will search for another doctor who will.

"Stress is a beast. I think it has caused you to have some mild depression. Let me prescribe a low dose of a medication to see if that will help."

"I bet you aren't sleeping well. Let's put you on something for a while to help you get some better rest. That should make a difference."

"You are likely perimenopausal. Let's do a low-dose birth control pill to try to regulate your hormones."

Those are just a few examples of what medical providers will typically offer people with similar stories. None of the choices are bad in and of themselves.

They just aren't getting to the root issue of what is going on. They are treating the symptoms, not the causes.

The topic of this book will be thyroid issues. I will mention other hormone systems and how they interact with the thyroid, but they will not be the primary focus.

After years of research, studying, talking to other medical providers, and trial and error, I believe that I have developed a strategy that better identifies thyroid issues and offers many more options to treat those issues once they are found.

This system isn't perfect. We are constantly learning more about the thyroid and other hormone systems. We need to be willing and able to incorporate new information into our treatment strategies.

I suspect that we will be treating thyroid issues somewhat differently in ten years from how we treat them now. For now, however, this is the best program that utilizes the latest information that we currently know.

If you have symptoms that you have always thought were caused by some kind of thyroid problem, there is a strong probability that you are right. Thyroid problems are everywhere.

The more I look for them, the more I find them.

Most textbooks or websites will say that hypothyroidism occurs in 5-10% of the population. When you dive into the studies used to get those numbers, however, an obvious problem shows up: How do they define hypothyroidism?

Most experts consider the TSH lab test to be the gold standard for diagnosing thyroid disease. A TSH above the reference range equals hypothyroidism. A TSH below the reference range equals hyperthyroidism.

For years, conventional medicine defined hypothyroidism as a TSH >10. A TSH level between 5 and 10 was defined as subclinical hypothyroidism.

Recently, however, many experts are saying that the upper limit of normal for the TSH should be much lower. That would likely make the percentage of the population with hypothyroidism higher than 5-10%.

One study even showed that up to 30% of people with a TSH >3 had an undiagnosed thyroid disease.

The Wickham Survey[1], which studied the thyroid levels of 2,779 randomly selected people from Wickham, England, from 1972 to 1973 and then followed them for the next 20 years, showed that anyone with a TSH above 2.0 had an increased risk for the development of hypothyroidism.

The NHANES III survey[2] screened 17,353 people from 1988 to 1994. They excluded anyone with a disease known to affect thyroid function. The results showed that about 3.7% of the population had a TSH >4.5. 95% of people had a TSH between 0.3 and 2.5.

The Framingham study[3] showed that 4.4% of people > age 60 had a TSH above 10.

The experts have been arguing ever since about what we should consider to be a normal TSH level.

I personally believe that there is sufficient data to suggest that any TSH >2.0 meets the criteria for hypothyroidism.

A valid argument could even be made that there is likely some degree of thyroid dysfunction if the TSH is above 1.0.

However, it shouldn't end there. The TSH is still valuable, but it is one of several thyroid tests that are available today.

Imagine only using 40 to 50-year-old information in other areas of your life.

Checking multiple thyroid tests will give us much more information than any single test can give (as I will discuss later in the book).

We have learned so much more about the thyroid over the past 50 years, and we are learning more constantly.

I believe we owe it to society to incorporate new information into our thyroid management of patients.

Just because we have always done something a certain way doesn't mean it is the best way.

That is the purpose of this book: Let's review what we know about the thyroid and compare it to what is considered standard of care for the diagnosis, treatment, and management of thyroid disease.

If some of the things we are doing are obsolete, or if new data shows there is a better way to do something, let's admit it and make the appropriate changes.

I truly believe that all medical providers want to do the best job that they can when taking care of patients. Part of that includes being open to new information and having a willingness to admit there may be a better way to manage something.

If you are someone who suffers from thyroid issues (or at least you think you may), then hopefully, this book will give you some real information that you can use to help yourself.

You will hopefully learn what questions to ask your medical provider, what lab tests to request, how to interpret those test results, which thyroid medications or supplements might help you, and so much more.

I recommend that you read through the book entirely at least once, then go back and re-read any chapters that were either confusing or more directly pertain to your current situation.

I hope this book can also serve as a reference for both patients and medical providers when they need help with a thyroid issue.

I would like to give a big shout-out to Dr. Westin Childs, who mentored me through much of my journey of learning thyroid management. His website, www.restartmed.com, is an invaluable resource for thyroid blog articles and high-quality thyroid supplements.

Now, let's get started!

1.

WHY IS IT SO HARD TO GET A THYROID DIAGNOSIS AND OPTIMAL THYROID CARE?

"Judy," a pleasant but frustrated woman in her mid-40s, came to see me in my office recently. She was desperate for help. For the past several years, she had felt progressively worse—always tired, constipated, constantly "cold," unable to lose weight, and gradually losing her hair, just to name a few of her symptoms. Judy said, "I am convinced that I have a thyroid issue, but no one ever finds anything wrong." She had seen multiple doctors but had always been told that all of her labs were normal.

After listening to her discuss her multiple symptoms and expressing her severe frustration with the medical system to that point, I tried to lighten the mood. "Wow! Other than that, Mrs. Lincoln, how was the play?" She laughed and seemed to relax a little bit. We completed her medical history and physical exam, and I ordered a complete lab workup for the next day. A few days later, her results showed up in my inbox. Based on her complete thyroid panel results, she had obvious Hashimoto's thyroiditis and hypothyroidism. When I talked to her about the results, she began crying and said, "I don't understand. Why hasn't this been found before now? I have been begging for help for so long." Within a few weeks of starting my thyroid treatment program, she started feeling better than she had in years.

I would love to tell you this story is rare. Unfortunately, I see it on a regular basis.

Thyroid management was one of the easiest subjects in my medical training. As a medical student and resident, I was taught that you only need to monitor the thyroid stimulating hormone (TSH) lab test.

If it is in the normal range, there is no thyroid issue to address. If it is low, the patient has hyperthyroidism, and you need to refer them to an endocrinologist. If it is high, the patient has hypothyroidism, and you need to start them on Synthroid (levothyroxine).

I was taught that there was no need to check any other lab tests. Even if the thyroid antibodies were elevated, there really wasn't anything you could do about it, so, no need to check them. Easy as can be.

In fact, that is exactly the current thyroid treatment paradigm recommended by the American Thyroid Association.[1]

There are three main components to their recommended thyroid treatment:
- The TSH is the single best screening test for primary thyroid dysfunction for the vast majority of outpatient situations.
- T4 is converted to T3 easily as the body needs it. Therefore, levothyroxine is the only thyroid medication that is needed.
- A normal thyroid state is present if the TSH is within its reference range.

There is much more to it than that for most thyroid patients. I suspect that most medical providers intuitively realize this is true purely based on how many thyroid patients are unhappy with their current thyroid management.[2]

The thyroid hormone system is extremely complex and requires much more understanding to diagnose what is going on in each specific situation and to design a treatment program that will help the problem.

Thyroid function is regulated at so many different levels, is impacted by so many different systems, and requires the optimal function of other organ tissues to operate normally.

Dysfunction in any of these areas can cause symptoms and problems that simply will not be detected by standard TSH testing, and treating those patients with only levothyroxine will not get most of them to an optimal state.

Why is there such a disconnect in medicine? Why are so many people living with undiagnosed and untreated or undertreated thyroid issues? We need to look at the history of how mankind has diagnosed and treated the thyroid over the centuries to get a better answer to these questions.

TIMELINE OF THYROID DIAGNOSIS AND TREATMENT

Ancient Greece	Afflicted people consumed marine sponges and/or seaweed to treat their swollen neck glands.
13th Century	De Villanova noticed that sponges only cured goiters that were in young people. Little to no effect on large, chronic goiters.
1789	Association between goiter and cretinism was identified.
1811	Courtois noted a purple vapor arising from seaweed ash. Gay-Lussac subsequently identified it as iodine, a new element.
1813	Coindet hypothesized that seaweed and sponges helped with goiter because of their high iodine content.
1819	Straub proved that marine sponges are rich in iodine.
1830s	Boussingault advocated giving iodine-rich salt to prevent goiter.
1848	Sir Robert Graves first described patients with hyperthyroidism (what we now call Graves' Disease).
1869	5000 French children with goiters were treated with iodine tablets. 4000 of them were cured or improved.
1883	Semon suggested that myxedema was due to thyroid insufficiency after seeing patients develop myxedema after having their thyroid removed.
1893	British physicians successfully treated myxedema with injections and/or oral doses of animal thyroid extract.

1916	Dr. David Marine began iodine prophylaxis studies in the US.
1922	Switzerland began a national iodized salt program.
1924	Wide use of iodized salt began in the US.
1925	T4 was identified and given in IV form.
1950s	Commercial T4 and T3 became available.
1950-1970	Patients treated with thyroid medication were found to have a higher rate of cardiovascular disease and death.
1970	It was discovered that 80% of T3 is converted outside of the thyroid gland.
1971	TSH RIA lab test became commercially available. TSH suppression (lowering the level) was found to predict the risk for cardiovascular disease.
1972	T3 RIA lab test became commercially available.
1973	T4 RIA lab test became commercially available.
1984	JAMA declares that natural desiccated thyroid (NDT) medication is "obsolete."
Prior to 1985	NDT was produced based on its iodine content, NOT its thyroid hormone content.
1985	NDT production became standardized based on its thyroid content. Cardiac deaths in patients taking it plummeted.

DEFINITIONS:

The timeline contains some medical terms that are likely foreign to you. The common terms that we use today (hypothyroidism, Graves' Disease, Hashimoto's, etc.) have really only been used over the past 100 years. Prior to that, the following terms were used for what we now know are thyroid diseases:

- **GOITER** – Enlargement of the thyroid gland. It typically presents with swelling in the neck.

  It is sometimes even painful.

  Iodine is an element that is essential for life. We can't produce it ourselves, so we must consume it regularly in our diet.

  The thyroid is the only part of the body that can absorb iodine. When the body is iodine deficient, the thyroid gland will enlarge to try to absorb more of it (what we call a goiter).

  Goiters are more rare today because of iodine supplementation but are still seen quite often in lesser degrees.[3]

- **CRETINISM** – We now know this was due to chronic iodine deficiency or the congenital lack of thyroid hormone production. These people had short life spans, short stature, swollen faces, and limbs, bone issues, and were typically cognitively slow.[4]

- *MYXEDEMA* – It resembled cretinism in many ways, but it was only seen in adults, typically women. It caused a swollen face, slowness of thought and movement, feeling cold, severe dry skin, and atrophy (shrinkage) of the thyroid gland.[5]

WHAT CAN WE LEARN FROM THIS MELINE?

Like many institutions in the world, the medical establishment is huge, set in its ways, and often unyielding. It takes years to form a consensus on accepted treatments for conditions. Once that consensus is formed, it is even harder to change it.

Studies have shown that once a medical discovery has been found, it typically takes an average of **17 years** before it is incorporated into regular medical treatment protocols.[6] That is similar to what has happened with the diagnosis and treatment of thyroid issues.

Prior to 1970, thyroid conditions were mostly a clinical diagnosis; there was little or no lab testing to confirm whether the doctor's clinical suspicions were correct. The diagnosis was made based on the symptoms and physical exam of the patient.

Thyroid medication was then given, and the patient response was gauged purely by how much their symptoms improved and/or what side effects they developed.

Many of these patients were obviously getting excessive doses of thyroid medication. This put a big strain on their hearts and led to an increase in cardiovascular deaths.

As my mom would often say, "You're cutting off your nose to spite your face." In other words, we were solving one problem but creating another one.

In 1971, laboratories developed an affordable way to measure TSH levels accurately and quickly. Doctors finally had a way to truly measure a patient's thyroid hormone level!

They learned that patients with low (suppressed) TSH levels had higher levels of heart issues. The standard of care in medicine, therefore, became to not suppress TSH levels in thyroid patients to prevent heart issues from occurring.

Prior to 1985, natural desiccated thyroid (NDT) medication was produced based on its iodine levels, not its thyroid hormone levels. As a result, there was a wide variance in thyroid doses in each bottle produced.

A patient might be getting an excessive dose of thyroid hormone when they only needed a much lower dose to control their hypothyroidism. This no doubt resulted in multiple cases of drug-induced hyperthyroidism, which increased cardiac issues.

Doctors, therefore, began using synthetic T4 (Synthroid) instead of NDT. It provided a more consistent, reliable dose.

In 1984, the Journal of the American Medical Association (JAMA) even made the statement that the use of NDT medicine should be considered "obsolete."[7]

That sounds great and makes complete sense. There are, however, some problems with this plan: We have learned much more about the thyroid and how to make thyroid medication since that time.

WHAT DOES THE THYROID DO?

Most people have a general idea about the thyroid gland, but let's look a little deeper into what functions it really controls:

- **Plays a major role in metabolism/metabolic rate** – When the thyroid gland is under-functioning, the rate at which calories are expended drops.
- **Supports normal heart function/heart rate** – Excess thyroid hormone can cause heart palpitations and even increase the risk for atrial fibrillation. Low thyroid hormone can lead to a slow heart rate (bradycardia) and increase the risk of congestive heart failure.
- **Regulates digestion** – Thyroid hormone has a direct effect on the movement of food/wastes in the digestive tract (called peristalsis). Low thyroid hormone often leads to problems with constipation.
- **Improves brain function/activates the neurological system** – Low thyroid hormone regularly causes symptoms of brain fog and reduced cognition.
- **Regulates reproductive system/menstrual cycle** – Abnormal thyroid function commonly causes a disruption in the menstrual cycle and can lead to infertility.
- **Regulates bone density** – The thyroid gland produces calcitonin, which regulates calcium levels and bone mineral deposition. Low thyroid function can lead to elevated serum calcium and bone loss.

Obviously, the thyroid gland is essential for optimal health. You will not reach your optimal level of health until your thyroid function is optimized.

HYPOTHYROIDISM

By far, the most common thyroid disorder is a low thyroid hormone level, which is called hypothyroidism.

Simply put, hypothyroidism is everywhere.

Most medical associations state that up to 10% of adults in the US have hypothyroidism. In my experience, that estimate is low.

As I will discuss in detail later in the book, there is some disagreement about what constitutes hypothyroidism.

If you use my recommended criteria and lab values to diagnose hypothyroidism, the number of adults with hypothyroidism is probably closer to 30-40%, in my experience.

Hypothyroidism is more common in women.

Most hypothyroidism (~90%) is caused by Hashimoto's thyroiditis, which I will discuss in detail in Chapter 5.

Hypothyroidism is commonly found in other autoimmune diseases. In fact, it is recommended that someone with any autoimmune condition have their thyroid labs checked periodically.

Thyroid hormone is essential for normal growth and development. Because of this, all infants in the US are screened for congenital hypothyroidism.

COMMON HYPOTHYROID SYMPTOMS

What are the most common symptoms of hypothyroidism?

Here are the ten most common:

1. Fatigue, even after sleeping 8-10 hours at night or needing to take a nap daily.
2. Weight gain or inability to lose weight.
3. Mood issues such as mood swings, anxiety, or depression.
4. Hormone imbalances such as PMS, irregular periods, infertility, and low sex drive.
5. Muscle pain, joint pain, carpal tunnel syndrome, or tendonitis.
6. Cold hands and feet, feeling cold when others are not, or having a body temperature consistently below 98.5 degrees.
7. Dry or cracking skin, brittle nails, and excessive hair loss.
8. Constipation.
9. Mind issues such as brain fog, poor concentration, or poor memory.
10. Neck swelling, snoring, or hoarse voice.

If you have five or more of the above symptoms, there is a strong likelihood that you have hypothyroidism.

Keep in mind that most hypothyroid symptoms are nonspecific, meaning that a multitude of other disease states could cause them. For this reason, lab testing should be performed to confirm or rule out the presence of hypothyroidism.

Did you notice the wide variety of the symptoms? Why is that?

Every cell in the body has a thyroid receptor.[8] Whichever cells are not getting enough thyroid hormone will determine what symptoms you may have.

For instance, if your brain is deficient in thyroid hormone, you may have symptoms of brain fog or memory loss.

If your skeletal muscles are lacking thyroid hormone, you may have chronic pain or tender points.

If your gastrointestinal tract is low in thyroid hormone, you may have constipation or other GI-related symptoms.

Studies have shown that age, gender, existing disease, and certain medications can all impact thyroid hormone conversion in the body.[9]

Just for completeness, there are numerous other symptoms that can be caused by hypothyroidism, many of which are listed on the next page.

SIGNS AND SYMPTOMS OF HYPOTHYROIDISM

- Fatigue
- Lethargy
- Low endurance
- Slow speech
- Slow thinking
- Poor memory
- Poor concentration
- Depression
- Nervousness
- Anxiety
- Worrying
- Easy emotional upset
- Obsessive thinking
- Low motivation
- Dizziness
- Sensation of cold
- Cold skin
- Decreased sweating
- Heat intolerance
- Non-restful sleep
- Insomnia
- Thick tongue
- Swelling of face
- Sparse eyebrows
- Low basal activity level
- Low basal temperature
- Slow resting pulse rate
- Long-normal intervals on ECG
- Swelling of eyelids
- Dry skin
- Dry mucous membranes
- Constipation
- Unexplained weight gain
- Paleness of lips
- Shortness of breath
- Swelling
- Hoarseness
- Loss of appetite
- Prolonged menstrual bleeding
- Heavy menstrual bleeding
- Painful menstruation
- Low sex drive
- Impotence
- Hearing loss
- Rapid heart rate
- Pounding heartbeat
- Slow pulse rate
- Pain in the front of the chest
- Poor vision
- Weight loss
- Wasting of tongue

- Indistinct or faint heart tones
- Low QRS voltage on ECG
- Emotional instability
- Choking sensation
- Fineness of hair
- Hair loss
- Blueness of skin
- Dry, thick, scaling skin
- Dry, coarse, brittle hair
- Paleness of skin
- Puffy skin
- Puffy face or eyelids
- Swelling of ankles
- Coarse skin
- Brittle or thin nails
- Dry ridges on nails
- Difficulty in swallowing
- Weakness
- Vague body aches and pains
- Muscle pain
- Joint pain
- Numbness or tingling
- Protrusion of one or both eyeballs
- Brain fog
- Cardiac enlargement on x-ray
- Fluid around heart

It is obviously not necessary to have every symptom listed. Just know that the more symptoms you have, the higher the likelihood that you have hypothyroidism.

CAUSES OF HYPOTHYROIDISM

So why does our thyroid stop working normally in the first place?

The causes of hypothyroidism are typically classified as primary, secondary, tertiary, and peripheral.[10]

1. **Primary** – These account for over 95% of hypothyroidism.

Basically, something has directly damaged the thyroid gland, preventing it from producing normal amounts of thyroid hormone.

By far, the most common reason is autoimmune thyroiditis (also known as Hashimoto's thyroiditis and often I will refer to it simply as Hashimoto's). Some experts suggest that up to 90% of all hypothyroidism is due to it.

I will discuss Hashimoto's in much greater detail in Chapter 5, but for now, just think of it like this: Something has triggered your immune system to make antibodies against parts of the thyroid gland.

Genetics and environmental factors appear to play a role. Things such as too much iodine, selenium deficiency, vitamin D deficiency, and moderate alcohol use all appear to increase the incidence of Hashimoto's.

The thyroid antibodies slowly destroy the thyroid until it reaches a point where it cannot produce enough thyroid hormone. Hypothyroidism results.

Other causes of primary hypothyroidism include iodine deficiency, surgical removal of the thyroid, damage to the thyroid from other neck surgeries or injuries, and post-radioactive iodine ablation of the thyroid.

Rarely there can be genetic mutations that prevent normal thyroid production, or the thyroid hormone molecule itself can be abnormally shaped, which prevents it from attaching to thyroid receptors.

There are also some medications that block normal thyroid function. These include thalidomide, some monoclonal antibodies, antiepileptic drugs, amiodarone, and lithium.

2. Secondary – These are due to problems with the pituitary gland.

Typically, surgery, radiation treatment, or a pituitary tumor has caused an impairment in TSH production. Without TSH stimulation, the thyroid gland reduces or even stops thyroid hormone production.

3. Tertiary – These are due to problems with the hypothalamus.

Again, either a tumor in the hypothalamus or damage from surgery or radiation causes TRH production to drop or stop. This leads to the cascade of low TSH secretion by the pituitary and low thyroid hormone production by the thyroid gland.

4. Peripheral – These are rare conditions, typically genetic. Either there is an overproduction of deiodinase 3 (which inactivates thyroid hormone), or there is a receptor defect that prevents thyroid hormone from binding normally to the thyroid receptors.

Knowing the cause of your hypothyroidism is important to guide your medical professional on the best treatment plan.

If it is due to autoimmunity, there are some lifestyle changes and supplements that can slow or even reverse the condition, which we will explain in Chapter 5.

If you have a pituitary tumor, obviously, that will need to be addressed. There are likely other hormonal abnormalities that will need treatment.

If you are on a drug that is impairing your thyroid, then changing to a different medication could be the only treatment needed to correct your thyroid issue.

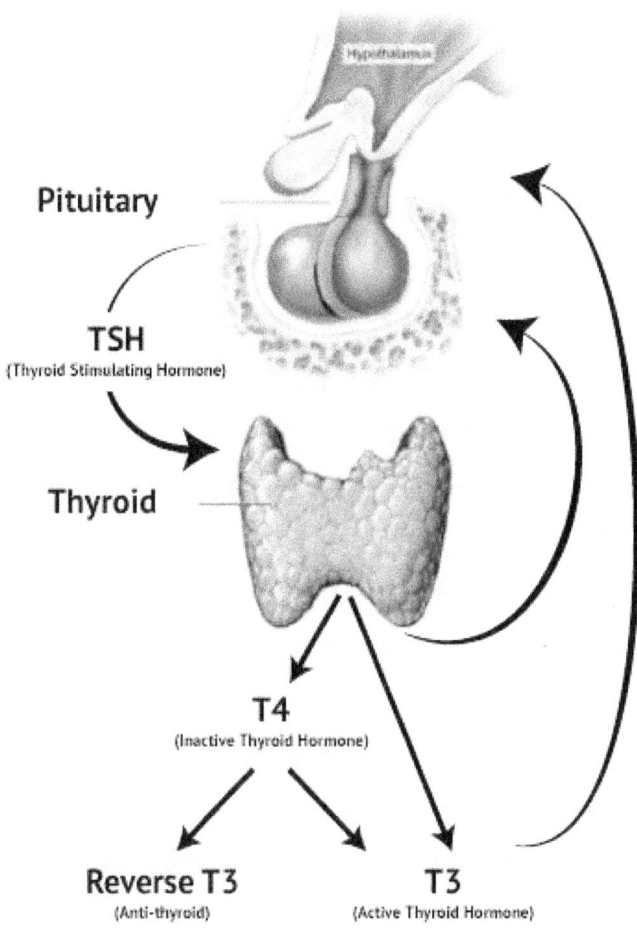

THE THYROID HORMONE SYSTEM IS EXTREMELY COMPLEX

Let's look at the thyroid cascade diagram. TRH from the hypothalamus stimulates TSH from the pituitary gland, which stimulates the thyroid gland to produce T4, which then converts to T3, which performs the needed thyroid functions in the cells of the body.

Pretty straightforward, right?

While those steps are true, we are learning there is much more complexity to the system than that.

Science has discovered that thyroid hormone levels in the body are highly regulated by enzymes called **deiodinases**.[11]

These enzymes control the thyroid hormone levels in the cells and bloodstream by either activating or inactivating them, depending on what the body or cells need at that time.

T4 circulates in the bloodstream to target tissues such as your liver, kidneys, muscles, heart, brain cells, skin, and so on.

Think of T4 as the transport form of thyroid hormone. It has little to no activity itself.

T4 can either be activated by converting it into the active hormone T3 or deactivated by converting it into the inactive metabolite, reverse T3. Which one occurs depends on what is going on in the body at that time.

T3 activates, reverse T3 deactivates.

For example, if you are exercising, active T3 conversion will occur in large amounts in your muscles, while reverse T3 conversion may occur in your intestines (you don't need to digest food while exercising).

Or if you are studying, you need more thyroid hormone in your brain cells, so T3 conversion will increase in your brain, while reverse T3 production in your muscles will increase (you don't need more muscle function while sitting at your desk).

Deiodinase enzymes are responsible for this activation and deactivation, both for the whole body and at the individual cellular level. The amount of T4 and T3 feedback to your hypothalamus influences how much TRH is released.

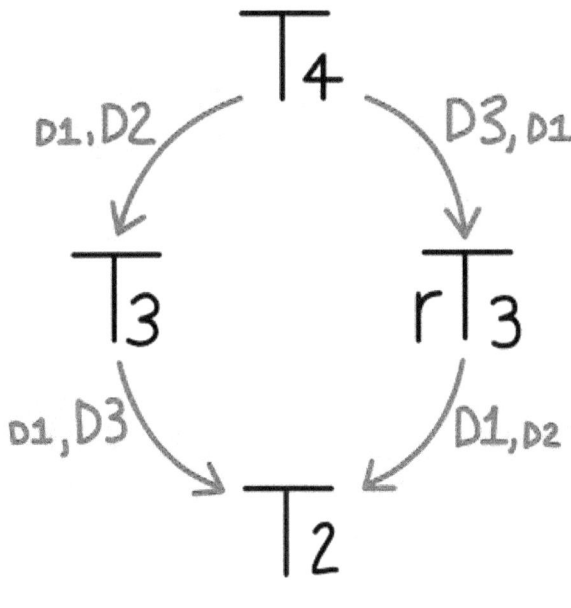

Three types of deiodinase enzymes have been discovered:

1. Deiodinase 1 (D1) – This functions as an "activating" thyroid enzyme. Its primary job is to convert T4 into active T3 in the peripheral cells of the body. It has very little activity in the pituitary gland, where TSH is produced. Overall, it is responsible for about 30% of all T3 production.

D1 is very sensitive to physical and emotional stress. The presence of things such as insulin resistance, leptin resistance, depression, diabetes, autoimmunity, dieting, and environmental toxins will suppress D1 activity and result in lower T3 levels.

D1 is also the primary enzyme that breaks down reverse T3 into T2.

2. Deiodinase 2 (D2) – This is another "activating" thyroid enzyme. Similar to D1, its primary job is to convert T4 into active T3. It is the main deiodinase found in the pituitary gland, so its activity has a direct effect on how much thyroid hormone is produced in the body. It is responsible for about 70% of all T3 production.

Unlike D1, D2 activity increases when the body is under physical or emotional stress. This can cause the T3 levels in the pituitary gland to be higher than the levels in the rest of the body. This can produce a normal TSH level even though the thyroid hormone level in the rest of the body is low.

D1 works mainly in the peripheral tissues, while D2 works mainly in the pituitary.

3. Deiodinase 3 (D3) – This is an "inactivating" thyroid enzyme. It converts T4 into the inactive reverse T3 and stimulates the breakdown of T3 into the less active T2 form. Many conditions cause your body to increase D3 function while down-regulating D1 and D2 function. This, in effect, shuts down or at least greatly reduces thyroid function in the body.

Why in the world am I mentioning these enzymes? Because **most medical providers don't understand or take into account the role of deiodinases in thyroid hormone function.**

THE T4-ONLY FALLACY

The prevailing thought in medical circles when it comes to thyroid management is to assume that the body does the T4 to T3 conversion process perfectly without any issues or problems.

If a patient is deficient in thyroid hormone (based on an elevated or higher than normal TSH level), then giving them more T4 in the form of levothyroxine will fix the problem.

Many times, this simply isn't true.

Were you diagnosed with hypothyroidism, given levothyroxine, and felt little or no improvement? I see it all the time.

So, what is really going on? Why does T4-only medication not help so much of the time? It all goes back to those deiodinase enzymes.

There are many common medical conditions that either deactivate or inhibit the function of the deiodinase enzymes. Here are just a few:

- **Inflammation**[12] – Inflammation inhibits D1 activity, which reduces T4 to T3 conversion.

- **Euthyroid Sick Syndrome**[13] – Decreases D1 and D2 activity and increases D3 activity. This results in a low free T3, high reverse T3, and normal TSH. This can occur with acute illness, chronic illness, and even dieting.

- **Gut Dysbiosis (leaky gut)**[14] – Having the wrong balance of bacteria in your gut can lead to elevated levels of lipopolysaccharides (LPS). LPS suppresses D1 activity, which impairs T4 to T3 conversion.

- **Dieting and Fasting**[15] – Fasting and restricting calories have been shown to decrease deiodinase activity, probably as a protective response to keep the body from burning excess calories.

- **Selenium Deficiency**[16] – This mineral is required for normal deiodinase activity. A deficiency of it suppresses D1 and D2 function and thus reduces T4 to T3 conversion.

- **Insulin Resistance**[17] – Insulin resistance has been linked to the production of abnormal deiodinase enzymes, which affects their function.

- **Obesity**[18] – Obesity is typically associated with insulin resistance, inflammation, and gut dysbiosis. All impair D1 activity, which reduces T4 to T3 conversion.

Studies have shown that deiodinase activity is even more important than the circulating levels of thyroid hormones when it comes to maintaining thyroid function in the body.

Even if your total thyroid hormone levels are low, your body can maintain decent cellular function and metabolism by increasing the amount of deiodinase enzymes available to convert whatever amount of T4 is available into active T3.[19]

Many people have normal T4 levels, but because of other medical conditions, poor diet, and other problems, their deiodinase enzyme activity is low or suppressed. As a result, they struggle to convert T4 to T3. The T4 instead converts mostly to reverse T3.

Since D2 activity is not as sensitive to these conditions as D1 activity, the TSH results and T4 results (which are the only ones most doctors check) will likely be normal, but the cells of their body are in desperate need of more T3.

They then develop all the typical symptoms of low thyroid that we discussed.

Here is the typical picture occurring in medical offices multiple times every day: A patient goes to see their doctor complaining of hypothyroid symptoms. The doctor checks a TSH (and maybe a T4 level). The levels are in the "normal" range, so instead of giving a thyroid medication (which they need), they are diagnosed with a myriad of other conditions – depression, fibromyalgia, insomnia, allergies, etc.

Even if the patient convinces the doctor to prescribe them a thyroid medication, they give them a T4-only medication such as levothyroxine. The T4 in the medication is converted mostly into reverse T3 instead of active T3 because of other conditions that are present. This continues to suppress the thyroid function in the body, so they get little to no symptom Improvement.

Do you see the problem?

Using T4-only medication is simply not adequate for most patients with thyroid problems because of other issues that affect their thyroid function.

THE TSH ONLY FALLACY

The TSH is a great thyroid lab test. It does an excellent job at detecting the more severe thyroid issues.

But what does the TSH really tell us?

Thyroid Stimulating Hormone (TSH) is produced by the pituitary gland. Its purpose is to stimulate the thyroid gland to produce thyroid hormone.

If the body is low in thyroid hormone, TSH levels will increase to stimulate the thyroid gland to produce more hormone. If the thyroid level in the body is high, TSH levels will drop since the body doesn't need more thyroid hormone to be produced.

It seems like that would make it the perfect test to check for thyroid function, doesn't it? Unfortunately, it's just not that simple.

The TSH indicates how much thyroid hormone is present in the **pituitary gland**. That level can be very different from the level of thyroid hormone in other cells of the body.

Three different things (at least) could be going on that the TSH level will not detect:

1. T4 to T3 conversion issues
2. Thyroid receptor issues
3. Autoimmune thyroid disease (Hashimoto's)

If the TSH is very high or very low, then it is a useful screen for thyroid problems. If it is normal or near normal, it could be missing several things that are important to detect.

I find it a bit bewildering that the thyroid is the only hormone of all the pituitary-controlled hormones where the testing of the free hormone levels is not considered standard of care.

Testosterone, progesterone, estradiol, cortisol, growth hormone, and thyroid hormone are all regulated similarly by the pituitary gland and hypothalamus.

With every single hormone besides thyroid, the serum level of the hormone itself is the primary lab test used to monitor levels of the hormone being tested.

For example, if a doctor wants to check a patient's testosterone or estradiol level, they check those direct hormone levels. They may also check the FSH and LH, but not without also checking the direct hormone levels. If they wonder about cortisol levels, they check serum cortisol, not the ACTH level.

Why is the thyroid different?

Free T3 and free T4 levels should be checked (in addition to TSH) to assess thyroid function.

Plus, the additional testing of thyroid antibodies and reverse T3 can help identify the cause of the thyroid dysfunction, such as autoimmune thyroid disease, thyroid receptor issues, and T4 to T3 conversion issues.

There is nothing about this that should be controversial.

Only checking the TSH is inadequate to screen for and properly monitor most thyroid diseases.

HYPOTHYROIDISM AND THE GUT

It is also important to at least briefly mention the strong connection between thyroid function and gut health.

Poor gut health can suppress thyroid function and even lead to autoimmune disease such as Hashimoto's. Conversely, low thyroid function can lead to an inflamed gut, which is a primary cause of intestinal permeability (leaky gut).

Did you know that 70% of the immune tissue in the human body is in the gut?

This portion of the immune system is what we call GALT, or gut-associated lymphoid tissues. These tissues store immune cells such as T & B lymphocytes that produce antibodies against potential threats that are consumed.

There are several ways in which gut issues directly affect thyroid function in the body and vice versa.

1. Intestinal Permeability (Leaky Gut Syndrome)

The spaces between the cells in the stomach and intestinal lining are what we call "tight junctions." These spaces are normally impenetrable to foreign proteins such as bacteria, viruses, and fungi.

However, inflammation has been shown to increase the gap between these cells, which allows foreign proteins to pass through the tight junctions and enter the bloodstream.

The result is what we call intestinal permeability (leaky gut syndrome).

When leaky gut syndrome occurs, foreign proteins are able to enter the bloodstream that normally would not. The body mounts an immune response against these proteins.

Many of these foreign proteins resemble proteins that are a natural part of the body, such as components of the thyroid gland.

Even though the immune system is making antibodies against those foreign proteins, the antibodies inadvertently attack the proteins in the body that resemble them. This is what we call molecular mimicry and is felt to be a major cause of Hashimoto's Thyroiditis.[20]

Thyroid hormones have a direct influence on the tight junctions in the gut. Studies have shown that T3 and T4 protect the gut mucosal lining from stress-induced ulcer formation.[21]

Another study showed that patients with gastric ulcers had low T3 and low T4 levels and high levels of reverse T3.[22]

Also, thyrotropin-releasing hormone (TRH) and TSH hormones both influence the development of the GALT (Gut Associated Lymphoid Tissue).

The GALT is the largest mass of lymphoid tissue in the body. It consists of immune cells such as B and T lymphocytes, macrophages, antigen-presenting cells, including dendritic cells, and specific epithelial and intra-epithelial lymphocytes.

The role of GALT is to manage the immune response to all the antigens we are exposed to in the gut.

T4 also prevents the overexpression of intestinal intraepithelial lymphocytes (IEL), which are known to cause inflammation in the gut.[23]

2. T4 to T3 Conversion

Around 20% of T4 is converted to T3 in the GI tract. This conversion is directly related to healthy gut bacteria.

If there is an imbalance between pathogenic and beneficial bacteria in the gut, T4 to T3 conversion is significantly reduced.[24]

3. Cortisol

Inflammation in the gut raises cortisol levels. Cortisol decreases T3 levels while increasing reverse T3.[25]

4. Lipopolysaccharides (LPS)

Lipopolysaccharides are parts of the cell walls of intestinal bacteria. They negatively affect thyroid metabolism in several ways:[26]
- Reduce thyroid hormone levels
- Dull thyroid hormone receptor sites
- Increase reverse T3 levels
- Decrease TSH
- Promote autoimmune thyroid disease

5. Low Stomach Acid (Hypochlorhydria)

Low stomach acid increases leaky gut, inflammation, and infection.

Studies have also shown an association between chronic low stomach acid and autoimmune thyroid disease.[27]

6. Constipation

Constipation is a well-known, common side effect of hypothyroidism. Hypothyroidism causes this by slowing transit time (peristalsis).

Conversely, constipation can impair hormone clearance and cause elevation in estrogen, which in turn raises SHBG levels (see Chapter 2 for more information on SHBG). The higher SHBG levels bind even more thyroid hormone, which reduces free T4 and free T3 levels.

7. Gallbladder Dysfunction

A poorly functioning gallbladder interferes with liver detoxification and prevents hormones from being cleared from the body.[28]

Conversely, hypothyroidism impairs gallbladder function by reducing bile flow.[29]

All these connections make it clear that you can't have a healthy thyroid without a healthy gut, and you can't have a healthy gut without a healthy thyroid.

The first step should be to identify the cause of the gut dysfunction.

Possible causes include hypothyroidism, low stomach acid, infections, dysbiosis, food intolerances, stress, and more.

FINAL THOUGHT

I think it is important to make a quick comment before I continue.

Much of this book will be focused on the differences between current conventional thyroid treatments and how I believe thyroid issues should be managed. None of this is meant to be an attack on conventional doctors or medical providers and how they manage their thyroid patients.

Everything that we know about medicine we were taught in our training, or we learned through our own experiences and self-study.

My issue is with the current treatment protocols and medical societies and how resistant they are to incorporate the latest information about thyroid management.

The management of thyroid conditions has not significantly changed in the past 40 years. Would you accept using 40-year-old information and technology in any other area of your life?

SUMMARY:

• The thyroid is responsible for many bodily functions. These include metabolism, heart function, brain function, digestion, the reproductive system, and bone mineral maintenance.

• The thyroid system is extremely complex.

• Studies show that it takes an average of 17 years from the time of a medical discovery until it becomes standard medical treatment.

• The vast majority of medical professionals are taught to diagnose and treat thyroid issues based solely on the TSH lab test. That can miss many thyroid issues, including autoimmune thyroid disease, T4 to T3 conversion issues, and thyroid receptor issues.

• A complete thyroid panel is recommended for all thyroid patients. This includes TSH, free T4, free T3, total T3, reverse T3, TPO antibodies, and thyroglobulin antibodies.

• Treating hypothyroidism with levothyroxine is typically inadequate for most patients. This is usually due to other medical conditions that are also occurring, such as gut dysbiosis, inflammation, nutrient deficiencies, diet, and others. Changing to Tirosint, NDT, or adding T3 to the levothyroxine may be necessary for patients to get maximal improvement.

- Hypothyroidism causes literally hundreds of various symptoms. The most common include fatigue, weight gain, mood changes, constipation, hair loss, cold intolerance, and brain fog.

- The vast majority of hypothyroidism is due to autoimmune thyroid disease. Other causes include nutrient deficiencies, surgical removal, radioactive iodine treatment, and some genetic disorders.

- Discovering the cause of your hypothyroidism can help you and your medical doctor to tailor an appropriate treatment plan specific to your needs.

- Deiodinase activity is more important than the level of circulating thyroid hormones when it comes to maintaining normal thyroid function.

- Current thyroid management has not significantly changed over the past 40 years despite extensive new research and improvement in thyroid medication.

2.

THYROID LAB TESTS:
WHAT TO ORDER AND HOW TO
INTERPRET THE RESULTS

"Tonya" is a 61-year-old female who came to me for thyroid management. She had been diagnosed with hypothyroidism for over 20 years. Her primary care physician managed her thyroid prior to her visit with me. She was taking levothyroxine 0.1 mg daily. The dose had not been changed in many years.

The medication seemed to help when she first started taking it, but over the last several years, she noticed she was gaining weight, felt cold often, and was more tired than she would have liked. She mentioned it to her doctor, but she was told her thyroid test was normal, so no changes were needed. Over the past few years, she had also developed some hypertension, and her doctor told her she was a "borderline diabetic."

Tonya worked as an administrative assistant. She did not exercise regularly. She was not following any particular diet. Lab tests that I ordered showed a TSH of 2.78, free T4 of 1.03, free T3 of 2.9, reverse T3 of

19.7, negative thyroid antibodies, a 25-OH-vitamin D of 17.2, and a hemoglobin A1c of 5.9.

I instructed Tonya to eat a whole-food, low-carb, low-sugar diet. She was also instructed to walk for 15 minutes at least three days per week. I started her on ADK 10,000u daily for 90 days, then reduced to 5000u daily thereafter. I stopped her levothyroxine and instead prescribed NP Thyroid 60 mg daily. I also started her on a multivitamin containing iodine, selenium, zinc, adrenal adaptogens, and berberine 1 gm daily.

Three months later, Tonya returned to my office. She had a noticeable improvement in her fatigue, and she didn't feel as cole. She had started to walk "some" and was trying to reduce the sugar and carbs in her diet. Thyroid labs were improved, but her free T3 level was still a bit low at 3.2, her TSH was 2.45, her reverse T3 had dropped to 14.8, and her 25-OH-vitamin D was 53. Her NP thyroid was increased to 90 mg daily. She was instructed to look for any signs of hyperthyroidism, including sweat-ing, tremors, anxiety, or palpitations. She was scheduled to follow up in another three months.

Lab tests, in general, are incredibly valuable. They give us a glimpse into what is going on inside the body. Prior to the development of lab tests, doctors were completely dependent on the history and physical exam as their only tools to diagnose medical conditions.

Unfortunately, lab tests are far from perfect. They really only indicate what is going on in the blood and at an isolated moment in time.

What is happening in the cells (which is what we really want to know) may be **very different** from what is going on in the blood.

So, how do we know what is happening in the cells?

The only true way is to get a tissue biopsy! Since that is not going to happen except in very rare circumstances, we must do the best we can.

Checking serum (blood) levels is the next best thing.

HOW ARE LAB REFERENCE RANGES DETERMINED?

To better understand this topic, we need to discuss some basics of statistics (Oh, joy!).

When looking at something that occurs within a large population of people, the results will follow a predictable distribution across a graph.

For example, if you graph the heights of everyone in the world, the results will range from as little as 21.5 inches to as tall as 97 inches, with the average being about 68 inches. The majority of people in the world will be close to the average height. The further away from the average you go, the fewer people will be that height.

The result is what is commonly called a **Bell Curve:**

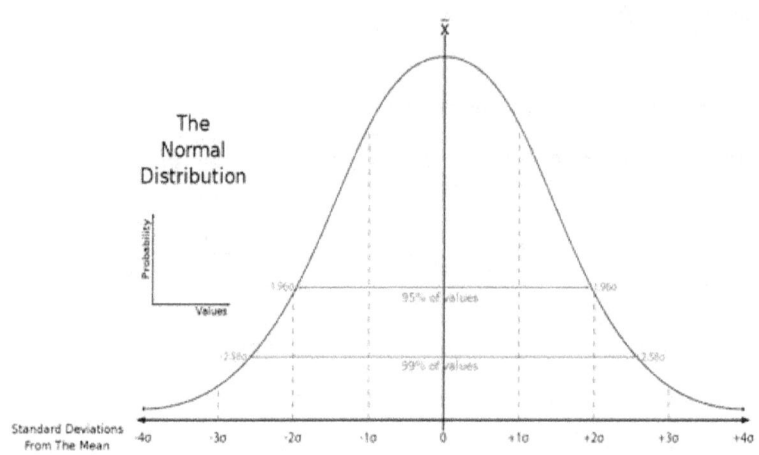

A Bell Curve produced by looking at a population assumes that everyone included in the graph is equivalent – same lifestyle, diet, medical history, etc. Any differences between the people will make the graph less accurate.

Determining the Bell Curve is how reference ranges for most lab tests are formulated. Any results falling within 95% of all results (2 standard deviations from the mean for you statistics nerds) are considered normal.

Overall, a Bell Curve is pretty accurate at determining where most results will fall on the graph. However, there are some problems with it.

Reference ranges do not always reflect a "normal" healthy population.

Health status, medications, supplements, stage of life, and hormone use are unknown, which can skew the range. Add in differences in lifestyles, physiology, dietary habits, and genetics, and it's even more difficult to define a normal population.

This is what happened when the reference range for the TSH lab test was first established.

It has since been shown that up to 30% of people with a TSH > 3.0 have undiagnosed autoimmune thyroid disease. This falsely skews the TSH range higher than it should be for a population with no thyroid issues.

When you take out that 30%, instead of a range of 0.4–- 5.0, it should instead be 0.4–- 2.0.

Some studies even argue that the upper limit should even be as low as 1.0.[1]

Thyroid Stimulating Hormone (TSH)					
TEST NAME	RESULTS	FLAG	REF. RANGE	UNITS	LOC
TSH	3.323		0.350 - 5.500	uIU/mL	PH

Studies have also shown that a TSH level >2.5 can indicate things such as metabolic syndrome.[2]

That is just one example of several.

THE DANGER OF LAB REFERENCE RANGES

A big problem with having "normal" reference ranges on lab results is it tends to make medical providers think the results are good as long as they fall within that range.

For years in my busy medical practice, I would often get multiple lab results back on several patients on the same day. Rather than study each result closely, I would typically scan each page looking for any result flagged as either "high" or "low." If they were not flagged, I assumed they were normal, and I paid no attention to them.

This certainly allowed me to detect results that were very abnormal, but there is no doubt that I missed some subtle trends that would have helped me diagnose and treat patients sooner.

My method was not unique. Every doctor that I have asked about it reviews their lab results the same way.

That is why **it is important for you to know the optimal ranges for your thyroid tests.** These ranges can be vastly different from the "normal" reference ranges listed from a laboratory.

Even if your doctor misses it, you can look at your own results and detect some underlying issues.

WHAT THYROID LAB TESTS DO YOU NEED?

A single thyroid lab test will only give us limited information about the thyroid function in the body. When several are grouped together, however, we can get a more complete picture.

That is why I recommend what I call the **complete thyroid panel**.

So much more information can be gleaned from these as a whole compared to only checking a TSH (typically the only one that doctors are taught to check).

The Complete Thyroid Panel includes:

1. TSH
2. Free T4
3. Free T3
4. Reverse T3
5. TPO Antibodies
6. Thyroglobulin Antibodies

THYROID LAB TESTS EXPLAINED

Okay, so you convinced your doctor to order all the tests in the complete thyroid panel. Now what? What do the results even mean? Let's discuss each of them in detail.

1. Thyroid Stimulating Hormone (TSH)— This is a hormone produced by the pituitary gland in the brain. Its purpose is to stimulate the thyroid (hence the name) to produce thyroid hormone. It is considered by most medical professionals as the "best" thyroid lab test.[3]

As a general rule, the TSH level is inverse or opposite of the thyroid hormone level in the body.

Let's look at the thyroid hormone cascade again that we discussed in Chapter 1.

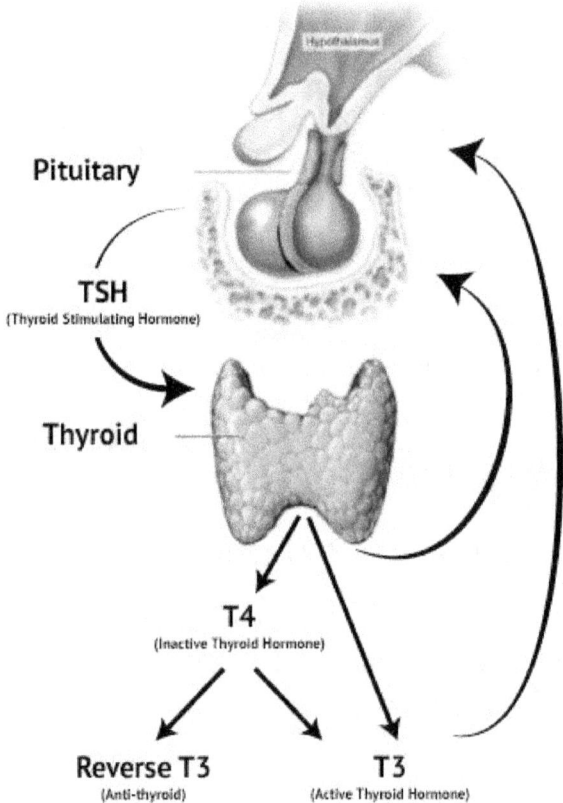

If there is a lack of T3 in the body, the pituitary will increase TSH production in the hopes of stimulating the thyroid to make more T3.

If there is too much T4 and T3 in the body, the pituitary will reduce or even turn off TSH production because the body doesn't need more thyroid hormone.

The TSH is an indicator of the amount of thyroid hormone present in the blood within the **pituitary gland.** This level is often different from the level of thyroid hormone within the cells of the body.

It does NOT give information on thyroid status in the peripheral cells, thyroid hormone conversion, or thyroid hormone cellular activation. That is why I strongly believe that TSH is not adequate by itself to monitor thyroid function and thyroid medication.[4]

If the TSH is substantially high or low, it is a good indicator of something going wrong in the thyroid gland. If it is normal or near normal, it doesn't tell us much just by itself.

Optimal Range = 0.3-1.0 uIU/mL

2. Free T4– A measurement of the amount of T4 hormone in the bloodstream that is not bound to a protein. T4 is much less biologically active than T3. To be activated, T4 must be converted into T3.

Think of T4 as the transport form of thyroid. It is a more stable molecule than T3, so the majority of thyroid hormone in the blood is in the T4 form. It is the **potential** activity of your thyroid gland.

A rise in free T4 levels would be expected in someone taking a T4-only medication. If they are taking a T3-containing medication, its levels will actually drop. The T3 in the medication suppresses T4 production by the thyroid gland. This is not dangerous but be aware that it may happen if you are on a T3-containing medication.

Optimal Range = upper ½ of the reference range (if not taking T3 medication)

3. Free T3— This may be the most important of all of the thyroid lab tests.

Free T3 represents the amount of circulating T3 in your blood that is **free** and **active** to do the work of thyroid hormone in the body and at the cellular level.

It can be low even when the TSH is in the normal range or even suppressed.

It is closely related to the metabolic function in thyroid patients and to their ability to lose weight.

Thyroid patients with a low T3 (even with a normal TSH) lose less weight and have more thyroid symptoms than someone with a higher free T3 level.[5]

The free T3 level has also been shown to be a more sensitive marker of non-thyroid illness than other standard lab tests.[6]

This is another reason why I believe it is so important to check regularly.

Optimal Range = 3.0-3.5 pg/mL (24 hours after taking T3-containing thyroid medication), 3.6-4-4 pg/mL (5-6 hours after taking T3-containing thyroid medication).

4. Total T3 - Total T3 is a measurement of the total amount of T3 in the blood, including that which is bound to protein.

The majority of T3 (and T4) in the blood is bound to proteins, which help stabilize the molecule. When they are bound, they are unable to enter cells and trigger their cellular functions.

Total T3 gives a better long-term view of the serum T3 levels when compared to free T3. It is particularly helpful when the patient is using a T3-containing medication such as NDT or Cytomel/liothyronine.

Like free T3, the total T3 is closely linked to energy production and the ability to lose weight.[7]

Optimal Range = upper 50% of the reference range

5. Reverse T3 - Reverse T3 is another test that is rarely ordered but gives vital information on thyroid function in the body.

T4 can either be converted into active thyroid hormone T3 or the inactive thyroid metabolite reverse T3. Which one it creates depends on the current needs of the cells in the body.

If your body has an immediate demand for more energy, more T4 will convert to T3. However, if your body wants to slow down metabolism, more of the T4 will convert into reverse T3. This system evolved to help your body closely regulate its energy use and production. Like all hormone systems, it can become dysregulated. That is when problems start arising.

Things like calorie-restricted diets, gut dysfunction, and inflammation can actively block T3 production and cause the reverse T3 levels to skyrocket.[8] Acute illness will also cause reverse T3 to rise dramatically, as will certain nutrient deficiencies (zinc, iodine, selenium, etc.). During those times, the body increases reverse T3 to slow the metabolism so that energy can be used to heal the body.

Unfortunately, the body tries to do the same thing with chronic illness and inflammation. It is just not as helpful because the result is typically weight gain and hypothyroid symptoms.

Optimal Range = <15 ng/dL

6. Thyroglobulin Antibodies and Thyroid Peroxidase (TPO) Antibodies - The tests measure the levels of two different antibodies that attack and damage your thyroid gland.

The presence of these antibodies in the blood indicates that your immune system is producing antibodies against your thyroid gland.

Most doctors do not routinely check these antibody levels because it is believed that their presence doesn't change the management of the patient.[9] I strongly disagree with this belief. Many autoimmune diseases can be reversed, especially if detected early.

Elevated thyroid antibodies can cause symptoms even when thyroid lab tests are otherwise normal.10

Tracking your antibody levels is a great way to monitor your disease state.

Keep in mind, however, that late-stage autoimmune thyroiditis (Hashimoto's) can result in so much damage to the thyroid gland that even the thyroid antibody levels will decline.

Optimal Range = TPO <35 IU/mL, Thyroglobulin Ab <35 IU/mL
The ultimate levels would be 0 for both, of course.

7. Sex Hormone Binding Globulin (SHBG) - This is a valuable test that can help you determine how active your thyroid is at the cellular level.

SHBG is a protein produced by the liver in response to two hormones: estrogen and thyroid.

If your estrogen is normal, SHBG can be used as a tool to monitor how well you are absorbing and using thyroid hormone at the level of the liver.[11]

If you have a low SHBG level from hypothyroidism, it **should** rise once you start taking a thyroid medication. If it rises, you can be assured that you are absorbing and utilizing your thyroid hormone adequately.

If you do not see a rise in SHBG after taking thyroid medication, you may need to reevaluate the dose and type of thyroid medication you are taking.

If SHBG gets too high, it can bind sex hormones such as testosterone and cause a whole spectrum of other problems. It can also mean that your thyroid medication dose is too high.

If it is excessively low, you are either deficient in thyroid hormone, or you may have some liver dysfunction.

Things like smoking and birth control pills can cause the SHBG level to be extremely high. In those cases, it is not a helpful tool for monitoring thyroid function.

Optimal Range = 50-70% of the reference range

8. Cortisol - Cortisol is the body's stress hormone. During times of high stress, cortisol levels will rise dramatically or sometimes even fall. In my experience, levels will eventually drop when stress occurs over a long period of time.

Many of the symptoms of chronic stress overlap with thyroid disease—fatigue, weight gain, anxiety, and many others. Even if you are on the proper treatment for your thyroid, if your adrenal system (which produces cortisol) is dysfunctional, you will not feel good.

Checking a morning cortisol level can function as a quick screen of your adrenal system. If it is in the normal reference range, it isn't really helpful.

However, if it is significantly above or below the reference range, that is a good indicator that adrenal dysfunction is likely present and needs to be addressed.

I recommend getting a morning cortisol level if you have chronic stress and severe fatigue as one of your primary symptoms.

If you get this test, make sure it is at 8:00 in the morning. That is when cortisol is at its peak level for the day. Checking it later in the day will make the results less reliable.

Optimal Range = 10-20 ug/dL

9. Thyroid Stimulating Immunoglobulins (TSI) - Just a quick mention about this test. If your initial thyroid tests show an extremely low (even zero) TSH level and if you are having symptoms of hyperthyroidism, you may need this test drawn.

TSI is the main test used to diagnose Graves' disease, also known as autoimmune hyperthyroidism.

Hyperthyroid patients are easily diagnosed when compared to hypothyroid patients, so this condition is rarely missed.

Their symptoms are usually quite severe—rapid weight loss, palpitations, tachycardia, tremor, anxiety, etc.

Optimal Range = As close to 0 as possible

10. T3 Uptake - You may see this test occasionally on thyroid panels that have been ordered by medical providers. I have not found it to be a particularly helpful test.

This test is used with total T4 levels to calculate a free thyroxine index (FTI).

It is an indirect measurement of binding proteins, the proteins in the bloodwork that bind to the majority of thyroid hormones in the bloodstream.

The results can be false in someone taking biotin, salicylates, corticosteroids, heroin, methadone, phenytoin, and perphenazine. Results can also be impacted by malnutrition, malignancies, kidney disease, and liver disease.

I generally don't recommend ordering this test. Stick with the complete thyroid panel. Normal ranges are typically 24-40%.

11. Free Thyroxine Index (FTI) - This test is used to indicate how much free T4 is in the bloodstream. It is calculated by dividing the total T4 by the T3 uptake.

Results can be affected by biotin and the other conditions mentioned under T3 uptake.

With the development of the free T4 test, there is really no need to order this test anymore.

Normal ranges are typically 1.2-5.0.

OPTIMAL RANGES FOR THYROID LAB TESTS

Lab Test	Abbr.	Normal Range (Lab Reference Range)	Optimal Range (Based on healthy adults)
Thyroid Stimulating Hormone	TSH	0.450-4.500 uIU/mL	0.3-1.0 uIU/mL
Free T4, Thyroxine	FT4	0.82-1.77 ng/dL	1.4-1.77 ng/dL
Free T3, Triiodothyronine	FT3	2.0-4.4 pg/mL	3.0-3.5 pg/mL
Reverse T3, Reverse Triiodothyronine	RT3	9.2-24.1 ng/dL	< 15.0 ng/dL
Total T3, Total Triiodothyronine	T3	71-180 ng/dL	150-180 ng/dL
Thyroid Peroxidase Antibody	TPO ab	0.0-34 IU/mL	0.0 IU/mL
Thyroglobulin Antibody	Tg ab	0-0.9 IU/mL	0.0 IU/mL

If you are checking your Free T3 levels 5-6 hours after taking your thyroid medication, the Free T3 level should be 3.6 - 4.4 pg/mL.

Remember, just because you get a lab result that is within the range of 95% of other people, that does not mean it is "optimal." It is important for you to know which lab tests to request but also to understand the results and be able to interpret for yourself how well your thyroid hormone system is working.

SUMMARY:

- There is a difference between a "normal" lab test and an optimal lab test. Your thyroid tests could be in the normal reference range, but you could still show evidence of thyroid issues.

- All thyroid patients should get a complete thyroid panel. This includes TSH, free T4, free T3, Total T3, reverse T3, TPO anti-bodies, and Thyroglobulin antibodies.

- You should know the optimal ranges for the complete thyroid panel so you can assess your own results and help guide your thyroid management.

3.

HOW TO ENSURE YOUR
LAB TESTS ARE ACCURATE

"Susan" came to my office for a yearly checkup. She was 48 years old and in good health except for hypothyroidism, which was diagnosed in her early 40s. Her only medication was NP Thyroid 60 mg every morning.

Overall, Susan was feeling great and had no complaints. When doing a review of her symptoms, she had no symptoms suggesting hypothyroidism or hyperthyroidism. Her mildly abnormal menstrual cycle was her only abnormal symptom. Her physical exam was unremarkable.

When her lab results came back a couple of days later, she had an unexpected result. While her TSH was an optimal 0.83, her free T3 level was 5.3. Reverse T3 was optimal, and thyroid antibodies were negative. Free T4 was 1.34.

When my nurse called her to discuss her results, she asked Susan if she had taken her thyroid medication the morning of her lab work. She confirmed that she had taken it "out of habit" about an hour before the labs were drawn.

We had her return the next day for repeat lab work and instructed her to wait to take her medication until after the labs were drawn. Those results showed a free T3 level of 3.5. I continued her current dose of thyroid medication, and she was instructed to follow up in six months for routine scheduled thyroid lab testing.

Obviously, you want your lab results to be as accurate as possible. You and your doctor simply can't make proper decisions about your treatment and thyroid medication dose if you don't have accurate results.

It's scary enough to primarily depend on a few simple lab tests to determine your best thyroid treatment plan. Making sure they are as accurate as possible is critical!

You may not realize that there are MANY factors that can negatively impact the accuracy of these labs, including when they are drawn, whether or not you are fasting when they are drawn in relation to when you took your medication, and more.

To push the odds in your favor, I recommend following these seven steps:

1. Get the complete thyroid panel.

In my experience, very few people ever get all of these lab tests drawn. Most people are surprised that there are thyroid tests beyond a TSH and a T4.

Why aren't all the tests checked? I discussed this in detail in Chapter 1. Basically, medical providers are simply not taught that they are important. Even if you convince them to order the proper tests, most medical providers don't know how to interpret them.

This is not a criticism of doctors or other medical providers; it is a criticism of the medical system as a whole. It is very set in its ways and very slow to adapt to new and changing medical treatments and research findings. That is why it is critically important that you know what tests to request from your doctor and how to interpret the results once you get them.

Here are the tests that I recommend: **TSH, free T4, free T3, total T3, reverse T3, TPO antibodies,** and **thyroglobulin antibodies.** If you are currently on thyroid medication, checking a **sex hormone binding globulin (SHBG)** can also be helpful. If you are under high physical or mental stress, a **morning cortisol** level should be checked as well.

It may not be necessary to order all the tests every time, but you should get the complete set as a BASELINE that you can use to compare with future tests.

If your current doctor is unwilling to work with you and order these tests, it may be time for you to seek out a doctor who is more comfortable with thyroid management. **Your health is at stake!**

2. Get fasting lab work.

Typically, medical providers do not think it is necessary to be fasting when thyroid labs are drawn. However, I disagree. Why? Because the consumption of food (including coffee) can impact the thyroid lab results.

Your thyroid controls the majority of metabolism in your body. Eating triggers your body to increase your metabolism. Your thyroid will, therefore, be more stimulated after you have eaten than if you are fasting.

In addition, food can interfere with the absorption of thyroid medication, which can change thyroid test results.

By the way, high cholesterol is an early marker of subclinical hypothyroidism[1], so you should periodically have your cholesterol panel checked as well (which requires fasting).

3. Check your labs BEFORE taking thyroid medication.

There isn't a complete consensus on the timing of taking your thyroid medication and when you should get your thyroid labs drawn.

After studying the research myself, I recommend getting your labs drawn about 24 hours after your last dose of thyroid medication.

Most people typically take their thyroid medication as soon as they wake up in the morning. On the day of your testing, just don't take your medication until after your labs are drawn. This 24-hour period marks the lowest that your thyroid level will be each day. That will help guide you and your doctor on whether your current thyroid medication dose is correct or if it needs to be adjusted.

Some experts recommend checking thyroid labs 5-6 hours after tak-ing thyroid medication. This would show the peak level of T3 in the blood (which should be 3.6-4.4 pg/mL). This would be helpful for someone who is extremely sensitive to T3 medication. Otherwise, I feel that getting the lab work around 24 hours after your last thyroid dose is accurate and more convenient for most patients.

This is really only important if you are taking thyroid medication with T3, such as NDT or Cytomel. The half-life of T4-only medica-tion is around 5-10 days. Holding it for 24 hours before getting your labs tested will have little to no effect on the blood levels.

4. Check your labs around 8:00 a.m.

This is not something that I have always recommended, but studying the research has convinced me of its importance.

Most hormones in the body PEAK first thing in the morning.

Thyroid hormone levels fluctuate throughout the day based on a number of factors—how awake you are, how active you are, whether you are ill, and many others. Because of this, it is important to have your thyroid labs checked around the same time of day each time so you can compare the results to previous tests.

If you have labs checked at 2:00 p.m. one day and then 8:00 a.m. the other, the results cannot really be accurately compared.

I recommend around 8:00 a.m. because that is also the time that cortisol levels peak. Cortisol and thyroid hormones work in tandem. Cortisol problems look very similar to thyroid problems, so checking both can help differentiate what is going on in your body.

If getting your labs drawn at 8:00 a.m. simply isn't possible, at least make sure they are drawn in the morning as close to that time as you can or reschedule for another day.

5. Avoid testing your thyroid on days 10-20 of your menstrual cycle.

Obviously, this is only important for women who are menstruating. Menopausal women and men do not need to worry about this.

If you have a fairly regular menstrual cycle, then knowing what day of the cycle you are on when you get your thyroid labs drawn can make a difference in the results.

Why is this important? During your menstrual cycle, estrogen and progesterone levels will fluctuate. Progesterone, in particular, can have an effect on thyroid hormone levels[2] so much that it can invalidate thyroid lab test results.

Since progesterone levels are highest during days 10-20 of the menstrual cycle, you should avoid getting your thyroid lab tests during those days. High levels of progesterone will improve thyroid test results, which could cause you and your doctor to think your thyroid levels are better than they actually are.

6. Avoid taking biotin prior to your thyroid labs.

Biotin is a nutrient that many people use to treat hair loss or help with hair growth. It is generally very safe and can be helpful. However, biotin can interfere with thyroid tests.[3] Biotin doesn't affect the thyroid function in the body but the lab tests themselves.

Biotin can make the thyroid lab results look more hyperthyroid than they really are. Someone with optimal thyroid function can look like they have hyperthyroidism, and someone who is hypothyroid can even look overmedicated.

It is best to avoid biotin for a few days before your lab tests to ensure that it doesn't interfere with the results.

Be careful because biotin can be in products such as multivitamins and hair growth products. It is common for people to take hair growth products because a frequent cause of hair loss is hypothyroidism.

7. Wait at least six weeks between lab tests.

Many thyroid patients who are anxious to feel better get their labs tested more frequently than the recommended six weeks.

The problem is it takes at least six weeks for your thyroid hormone levels to reach equilibrium. Testing earlier than that is just not useful and can even be harmful. It could cause the doctor to adjust your medication dose before your body has had a chance to reach that equilibrium state.

In addition, you are not likely to feel any better in such a short time. It can take weeks before the change in thyroid hormone level affects your clinical symptoms, even if you are on the proper dose of medication.

When it comes to treating your thyroid, you need to think in terms of MONTHS (not days or weeks). Changing supplements, medication doses, diet, and other things simply will not cause immediate results. It just takes time.

Summary:

- To ensure that your lab results are accurate, I recommend the following things:
  - ◊ Get a complete thyroid panel - TSH, free T4, free T3, total T3, reverse T3, TPO antibodies, and thyroglobulin antibodies.
  - ◊ Get your labs drawn around 8:00 a.m.
  - ◊ Get fasting lab work.
  - ◊ In most cases, get your lab work <u>before</u> taking that day's thyroid medication.
  - ◊ For females, avoid getting your thyroid labs drawn on days 10-20 of your menstrual cycle.
  - ◊ If you normally take biotin, stop it for a few days before getting your thyroid labs drawn.
  - ◊ Do not get your thyroid labs less than six weeks between medication changes.

4.

COMMON THYROID LAB PATTERNS TO HELP YOU IDENTIFY YOUR THYROID ISSUE

"Brenda" is a 42-year-old female who came to my office for a checkup. When I first asked her how she was doing, she said she was "fine." After I started doing a more specific review of systems, she admitted to several symptoms such as mild fatigue, hair loss, and weight gain of a few pounds over the past year despite not changing her diet or activity level. Her mother was diagnosed with hypothyroidism later in life.

"Doc, I'm 42 years old, I work full time, and I have three teenagers who are involved in multiple school activities. Of course, I'm a little tired."

Her physical exam was unremarkable.

Her lab results showed a TSH of 3.2, a free T3 of 3.2, a reverse T3 of 9.8, and normal thyroid antibodies. Non-thyroid lab results were unremarkable.

I explained to Brenda that she was showing some early signs and symptoms of hypothyroidism.

I prescribed a whole food, low-carb diet and a moderate exercise program that included yoga. I also started her on a multivitamin with selenium and adrenal adaptogens. We discussed stress management and proper sleep hygiene.

Brenda returned to my office three months later. She had incorporated everything I had discussed with her, and she was feeling better. Her TSH had dropped to 1.96. All other thyroid labs were optimal.

There are patterns of thyroid lab results that can indicate certain conditions that are going on in your body.

Most medical providers will not detect them because you can only see them if you have checked the complete thyroid lab panel. Since most medical professionals are only taught to check the TSH (and maybe a T4 level), the opportunity to gain insight into what is going on with the thyroid will be missed.

Why is detecting these patterns important?

Chronic medical conditions don't start overnight. They develop gradually over time. The earlier we can detect them, the better the chance of reversing them before they become severe.

For example, Type 2 diabetes can be completely reversed with diet and lifestyle changes if caught in the early stages. The longer a person has it, however, the more difficult and less likely it will be that the condition can be reversed.

The same is true for thyroid issues.

If someone has had Hashimoto's for 10 or 20 years, they likely have irreversible damage to the thyroid and will probably need thyroid medication for the rest of their lives.

If Hashimoto's is found early in the process, it is possible that lifestyle intervention and supplements could reverse it before permanent damage occurs.

So, let's look at some of these patterns:

1. Early Hypothyroidism

Instead of waiting until you have gained 20 pounds, are completely exhausted, or have lost a bunch of hair, wouldn't it be nice to detect your hypothyroidism BEFORE it gets to that point?

That is what we mean by EARLY hypothyroidism. It's the beginning stages of what will eventually become overt hypothyroidism with all the symptoms we discussed in Chapter 1.

People in this early stage typically have more subtle symptoms such as mild or moderate fatigue, mild hair loss, a few pounds of weight gain, etc.

If we can catch it earlier, we can prevent many of the more severe symptoms from occurring.

- *TSH* - Will be mildly elevated with any result greater than 2.0 uIU/mL. Most doctors will see the reference range listed on the results as being normal, up to 5.0 or even higher. Newer studies suggest that a TSH greater than 2.0 indicates a problem.
- *Free T4* - Low or normal (can be either)
- *Free T3* - Low or normal (can be either)
- *Reverse T3* - Normal
- *Thyroid antibodies* - Normal

With this condition, TSH is the most sensitive of the lab results to detect it. If your TSH is greater than 2.0, but your free hormones and thyroid antibodies are normal, it is time to act. Natural remedies that I will discuss throughout the book can help. Sometimes, even small doses of thyroid medication may be needed.

2. Thyroid Problems Related to Obesity

Obesity is a major problem for thyroid patients because of how the thyroid affects your metabolism.

Most people realize that low thyroid function (hypothyroidism) leads to weight gain, but you may not know that weight gain leads to low thyroid function.

This pattern looks like this:
- TSH - Low or normal
- Free T4 - Normal
- Free T3 - Low
- Reverse T3 - High or normal
- Thyroid antibodies - Normal

A LOW free T3 may be the only abnormality in this situation. If everything else is normal, but the free T3 is low, it is likely that the person's weight is affecting their thyroid function.

Reverse T3 may be normal at first, but it will eventually rise, and the free T3 will get even lower, especially in someone who is dieting or restricting calories or has lots of inflammation.

The more you diet and restrict calories, the higher the reverse T3 will rise. That is why it is so difficult to lose weight when you have hypothyroidism.

3. Thyroid Conversion Problems

These conditions refer to how well your body activates thyroid hormone by converting T4 into T3 (see Chapter 2).

The majority of people with thyroid issues have problems with thyroid conversion.

The lab pattern looks like this:

- TSH - Normal
- Free T4 - High or normal
- Free T3 - Low
- Reverse T3 - High
- Thyroid antibodies - Normal or high

These issues will be completely missed if you don't check ALL the thyroid lab tests. A TSH will be typically normal.

The free T3 and reverse T3 tests are the most important labs for identifying conversion issues. If the body has difficulty converting T4 to T3, it will instead convert the T4 to reverse T3. This typically causes hypothyroid symptoms and makes patients feel worse.

Conversion issues can be treated by taking T3-containing medication, addressing the underlying issue that is restricting the T4 to T3 conversion, lifestyle changes, and certain supplements.

4. Early Hashimoto's Thyroiditis

This refers to the stage in Hashimoto's thyroiditis where the thyroid is only slightly damaged. This damage is enough to likely cause some mild hypothyroid symptoms. Even though there is some thyroid damage, it is not yet enough to affect the TSH.

The result is most of the thyroid labs will be normal (or near normal), but the patient has hypothyroid symptoms, and the thyroid antibody levels (1 or both) will be elevated.

- TSH - Normal
- Free T4 - Normal or low
- Free T3 - Normal or low
- Reverse T3 - Normal
- Thyroid Antibodies - High (can sometimes be normal)

The key is to check BOTH thyroid antibodies (TPO and thyroglobulin). Either or both can be elevated.

If caught early, natural treatments may be enough to reverse the Hashimoto's (see Chapter 5).

NDT or T3 medication, however, is often needed to help treat symptoms and suppress antibody production.

Even if the TSH is normal, thyroid medication may be helpful in some cases. Low-dose naltrexone (LDN) and/or black seed oil can also be used to modulate antibody production.

This is a classic example of when asking about symptoms may be more important than lab results.

5. Low T3

Low T3 syndrome usually occurs because of chronic medical conditions.

If someone is in an accident or has an acute illness, the body responds to save energy so it can be used to fight the infection or treat the injury. It does this by reducing T4 to T3 conversion and increasing reverse T3 conversion.

This, in effect, shuts off or slows down the thyroid hormone's effect on metabolism. The medical term for this is *euthyroid sick syndrome.*[1]

This thyroid change works great in an acute setting. Unfortunately, it occurs quite commonly in a chronic setting as well, which isn't a good thing.

When your body is bogged down by one or several chronic medical conditions (diabetes, autoimmunity, obesity, etc.), the same reaction kicks in - low T3 conversion and high reverse T3 conversion. Since these chronic conditions don't typically resolve, the T3 conversion stays suppressed.

The lab pattern looks like this:
- TSH - Normal
- Free T4 - Normal
- Free T3 - Low
- Reverse T3 - High
- Thyroid Antibodies - Normal

The focus of this situation should be to treat the chronic conditions. When that occurs, the thyroid levels will often return to normal.

In some situations, giving thyroid medication (especially T3) can help speed up the recovery.

SUMMARY

There are several thyroid issues that can be detected by a complete thyroid panel, even before they have become a big problem. These can include autoimmune thyroid disease, obesity-related thyroid problems, early hypothyroidism, thyroid conversion problems, and low T3. Recognizing certain lab patterns can help you and your medical provider detect a problem, start treatment early, and potentially reverse the condition.

5.

HASHIMOTO'S THYROIDITIS

Andi is a 51-year-old female who came to the office complaining of pro-gressive fatigue, insomnia, constipation, and cold intolerance for the past several years. She had seen her PCP on numerous occasions, but her lab work was always normal.

She was still having monthly menstrual periods, but they were getting a bit more unpredictable. She was very strict with her gluten-free diet. She exercised regularly. Family history was positive for "thyroid problems" in her mother and sister.

Lab work was ordered, which showed a TSH of 4.7, free T4 of 1.14, free T3 of 2.8, reverse T3 of 13.2, TPO antibodies of 87, total testosterone of 3, FSH of 23, and estradiol of 118.
25-OH-vitamin D was 64, and vitamin B12 was 718. CBC and CMP were normal. AM cortisol was 6.2.

Andi was diagnosed with Hashimoto's thyroiditis, hypothyroidism, and perimenopause. She was prescribed adrenal glandulars and adaptogens, DIM, selenium, fish oil, and NDT Thyroid, and it was recommended that she consider testosterone replacement therapy. She chose topical testosterone cream that was compounded by her local compounding pharmacy. I also recommended that she remove dairy from her diet.

Her NDT thyroid medication was gradually titrated over the next few months until her symptoms were under control and her free T3 was above 3.5. TSH ultimately dropped to 0.358. Her energy, insomnia, constipation, and cold intolerance all greatly improved.

WHAT IS HASHIMOTO'S?

Hashimoto's thyroiditis is what is called an autoimmune disorder. Basically, your immune system goes rogue and starts attacking parts of your thyroid gland.

It was first described by a Japanese physician, Dr. Hakaru Hashimoto, in 1912. People in Japan consume large quantities of fish. Fish contain a lot of iodine, which we know in large amounts is a common cause of autoimmune thyroid disease.

Hashimoto's is the most common autoimmune disease in the US, and its incidence is rising rapidly.

When I was working in a full-time primary care medical practice, I typically diagnosed new cases of Hashimoto's on a weekly basis.

In other words, it's everywhere.

Up to 10% of the US population may have Hashimoto's, and it occurs more often the older we get. It is much more common in women. Seven women are diagnosed for every one man that is diagnosed.[1] It is more commonly seen around the time of puberty, pregnancy, and menopause, which seems to suggest that hormone fluctuations may play a role in the development of Hashimoto's. It appears to be more common in Caucasians and Japanese individuals.

CAUSES OF HASHIMOTO'S

No one knows definitively what causes Hashimoto's. We have a lot of evidence and scientific studies that may suggest certain things, but we just don't know definitively.

There appears to be a genetic predisposition that gets activated when exposed to certain triggers.

I can say from personal experience of treating thousands of patients that focusing on the areas I will discuss will result in improvement for most people.

This improvement may be seen as a decrease in thyroid antibodies, a decrease in overall inflammation of the body, or an improvement in how patients feel day to day.

From the perspective of the scientific and conventional community, there isn't a big rush to try to "figure out" Hashimoto's. They believe that autoimmune diseases are due to your genetics, and there really isn't a treatment that helps.

The current standard of care in conventional medicine is to treat any hypothyroidism caused by Hashimoto's with levothyroxine and adjust the dose as needed in the future as more of the thyroid gland becomes destroyed by the autoimmune disease.

I obviously strongly disagree with this position. I have seen patients improve after identifying root causes and removing as many of those causes from their lives as possible.

That said, here are the most **common triggers** that I see that cause or worsen Hashimoto's:

COMMON HASHIMOTO'S TRIGGERS

- Stress (physical, emotional, social)
- EBV infection
- H.pylori infection
- Nutrient deficiency (Vit D, zinc, selenium, glutathione)
- SIBO/SIFO
- Gluten sensitivity

1. Stress (emotional, physical, and/or social)

In my experience, stress is probably the single most important trigger of Hashimoto's. And by stress, I am referring to all types of stress.

Emotional stress - This stems from issues such as the inability to draw clear boundaries in your life or stress from the impact of relationships.

Physical stress - Excessive exercise, trauma, accidents, etc.

Social stress - This tends to be more mental in origin. It can include things like work stresses, crazy neighbors, etc.

It is clear that stress can have both a positive and negative impact on our bodies. It can be good if it's applied in a measured and calculated way.

For example, how many of us perform better at work if we have a lot of stuff to do or have a deadline to reach?

But once you tip the scales and it becomes excessive, the consequences in our body are profound. Many of my patients will start their story like this: "My health was great until _____." Fill in the blank with things such as "my divorce," or "I had pneumonia," or "my mother died," or "I had a bad car wreck," etc.

Whatever the stress was, it apparently triggered the genetic changes that resulted in the development of Hashimoto's.

I realize that identifying stress as the primary trigger may seem more frustrating than helpful. Many sources of stress can't be removed. You can't go back in time and not have the bad car wreck that started you down this path.

However, there are things you can do to improve how your body reacts to stress. Doing things such as meditation, adrenal supplementation, and improving sleep hygiene can be a huge help in reducing the severity and number of flares in the future.

2. EBV Viral Infection

Epstein Barr (EBV) is the notorious virus that causes infectious mononucleosis (mono). More and more studies are starting to link EBV with a multitude of diseases, including cancers and autoimmune diseases. It is part of the herpes virus family and is especially known to cause immune system issues.[2]

EBV is particularly good at evading our immune systems. And once we are infected with it, it is with us for life.

Over 90% of people worldwide have been exposed to EBV. While the vast majority of people have either an asymptomatic or only mildly symptomatic case, some people are affected much more severely.

Normally, our natural defense mechanisms will attack the virus and get it under control easily. However, if someone has issues such as poor nutrition, low vitamin D, and low CD8+ T cells, the virus may deplete our immune response, which results in a low-grade latent infection. This can result in the EBV virus taking up residence in various organs, such as the thyroid.

Our immune system continues to fight against the virus, which can result in antibodies being made against it that also harm the thyroid where it is residing. The result can be Hashimoto's.

In cases of latent infection, treating the patient with antivirals can have a positive impact on their Hashimoto's.

If the patient has only been exposed in the past but doesn't have signs of latent infection, then treating for an EBV infection will have little if any impact on their Hashimoto's.

3. H. pylori Bacterial Infection

H. pylori is a bacterial infection that can affect your immune system, kind of like EBV. Helicobacter pylori is well known by medical providers. It is a common cause of stomach ulcers.

For many years, researchers thought it took up residence in the stomach because of stomach ulcers. In actuality, we have learned that H. pylori is the cause of the ulcers, not the other way around.

This bacteria prefers to live in a low stomach acid environment. Anything that you are doing to your body to reduce the acidity in your stomach may create a breeding ground for this bacteria to thrive.

Once an infection has taken root, it gets into your stomach lining and causes inflammation in the stomach wall. This inflammation is likely why infections with H. pylori increase your risk of developing certain types of stomach cancer.[3]

But what H. pylori does to your immune system is more relevant to this discussion.

Infections with H. pylori have been implicated in triggering Hashimoto's and may also be associated with Hashimoto's flare-ups.

Thyroid patients tend to experience issues with low stomach acid due to their thyroid, which puts them at an increased risk of developing an H. pylori infection. When you add in the fact that so many people in the population regularly take acid-reducing medications, it's easy to see why H. pylori infections can be such a problem with thyroid patients.

The good news is, unlike EBV infections, H. pylori infections can be eradicated from the body. It may take multiple antibiotics in addition to other medications, but it can be done.

If you have Hashimoto's and also have any sort of intestinal issue such as acid reflux, heartburn, frequent nausea, etc., it is recommended that you be tested for an H. pylori infection.

There are blood tests and breath tests for H. pylori. You will need to see your medical provider to have these tests ordered and prescribed proper treatment if you are positive.[4]

It is also important to remember that H. pylori infections can return. If you have been treated in the past but are starting to have GI symptoms again, it may be time to be retested.

Blood tests for H. pylori only show if you have been infected in the past. They do not differentiate between old and active infections.

If you have a history of an H. pylori infection, you will need a breath test to see if you have an active infection.

4. Nutrient Deficiencies

Nutrient deficiencies do not cause Hashimoto's directly, but they create an environment that can make you more susceptible to other triggers.

Vitamin D – Vitamin D deficiency can impair your immune system, which makes you more susceptible to triggers such as stress and/or infections.[5]

Zinc – Zinc plays many important roles in thyroid function and immune function.[6] Zinc deficiency can impair immune function and impair T4 to T3 conversion.

Selenium – Selenium plays an important role in reducing thyroid gland inflammation. Selenium deficiency in itself may be a major contributor to the development of thyroid autoimmune disease. In fact, studies have shown that selenium supplementation can reduce thyroid antibody levels.[7]

Glutathione – Glutathione helps reduce thyroid gland inflammation and may be a helpful supplement in Hashimoto's.
Keep in mind that your body cannot produce glutathione if your selenium levels are low.[8]

5. SIBO/SIFO

The gut is the primary site of immune system regulation in the body. When you think about it, it makes sense.

The majority of our exposure to the outside world occurs on our skin (what we touch) and in our stomach and intestines (what we eat and drink).

Our gut contains an estimated 3-5 pounds of bacteria, which are essential for normal health. Collectively, we call these 100 trillion bacteria our **microbiome**.[9]

They communicate with our immune system, provide nutrients for our body, help manage our hormones, and much more.

When they are healthy, we are healthy. When they are unhealthy, we are unhealthy.

How we live and what we consume have a tremendous impact on the health of our microbiome.

Doing things such as eating processed foods, eating artificial sweeteners, living an excessively stressful life, taking prescription antibiotics, taking acid-blocking drugs, and more all negatively impact this vital community of bacteria.

A dysfunction of the microbiome can lead to opportunistic bacteria or fungus overgrowing in our gut. The conditions are called small intestinal bacterial overgrowth (SIBO) and small intestinal fungal overgrowth (SIFO).

This overgrowth can lead to immune dysfunction and inflammation, which can lead to the development of an autoimmune condition.[10]

Unfortunately, thyroid patients are already at an increased risk of developing SIBO due to a decrease in intestinal mobility.[11]

There are tests available to test for both SIBO and SIFO.

Most conventional medical providers have little to no experience with these conditions, so it may be necessary to see a gastroenterologist or functional medicine provider to get tested and treated.

Treating or normalizing your gut microbiome won't necessarily "cure" Hashimoto's, but I typically see significant improvement in Hashimoto's patients when their gut is improved.

6. Gluten Sensitivity

When it comes to gluten, there really is a spectrum.

On one end, you have people who have essentially zero reaction to gluten-containing food. On the other end are patients with celiac disease. They are severely allergic to gluten and will die if they continue to consume it.

Most people fall somewhere in between those two extremes.

Someone may have significant symptoms after consuming gluten, such as nausea, bloating, abdominal cramps, and diarrhea.

Others may have milder or non-GI symptoms that they may not even realize are due to gluten. These can include headaches, brain fog, joint pain, fatigue, anxiety, depression, and even skin rashes.

In my experience, most people have some degree of gluten intolerance/sensitivity.

Gluten can increase inflammation in the gut and in the body. This inflammation then causes problems in the lining of the gut, which leads to increased intestinal permeability, or what we call a leaky gut.

As the damage increases, bacteria and other foreign invaders enter the bloodstream, which triggers a strong immune response against them.

Many of these foreign bacteria resemble parts of our body. So, inadvertently, our immune system creates antibodies against parts of our body. This is called **molecular mimicry**.[12] An autoimmune condition may result.

It can be difficult to diagnose non-celiac gluten sensitivity.[13] However, it is so common, and gluten is such a common source of inflammation I typically recommend all thyroid patients do a trial of removing gluten from their diet.

Removing gluten from your diet for 90 days can dramatically improve your immune function and inflammation and doesn't cost anything to try.

Gluten-free recipes and other sources are readily available online.

STAGES OF HASHIMOTO'S THYROIDITIS

- Stage 0 – Genetic predisposition
- Stage 1 – Immune Cell Infiltration (+antibodies)
- Stage 2 – Subclinical Hypothyroidism (+antibodies, normal TSH
- Stage 2.5 – Thyroid Hormone Fluctuations
- Stage 3 – Overt Hypothyroidism (+antibodies, elevated TSH, low T4 and T3
- Stage 4 – Additional Autoimmune Diseases
- Stage 5 – End-stage Hashimoto's (decreased or negative thyroid antibodies)

STAGES OF HASHIMOTO'S

Not all Hashimoto's patients are the same. Some have mild symptoms, while others are completely riddled with debilitating symptoms.

Why the difference?

Much of it depends on the sheer amount of thyroid antibodies that are being produced. The higher the antibody level, the more inflammation and symptoms typically occur.

Some of it also depends on how long you have had Hashimoto's.

Let's look at the various stages of Hashimoto's and what is going on in each.

Stage 0 - When it comes to autoimmune diseases such as Hashimoto's, genetics play an important role in determining whether or not you will get a specific disease.

Stage 0 simply refers to a genetic predisposition for developing Hashimoto's.

Please realize that genetic predisposition is not an inevitability. It is simply a pathway you are at increased risk of following if you don't do some things to help prevent it.

More important than genetics are the triggers that I discussed in the previous section.

It is only when you combine a genetic predisposition with one or more of those triggers that you are primed to develop Hashimoto's.[14] If you have a family history of thyroid disease, Hashimoto's, or even other autoimmune diseases, you likely have an increased genetic risk of developing Hashimoto's.

Stage 1 - Immune Cell Infiltration (Positive Antibodies)

In this stage, immune cells infiltrate the thyroid gland. This results in inflammation.

Thyroid antibodies become detectable in lab work. Most people are still not diagnosed at this stage.

The symptoms associated with this stage tend to be very mild and nonspecific, so most patients don't realize it could be due to a thyroid issue. The symptoms may include slightly less energy or feeling a bit run down.

This is the best time to reverse Hashimoto's if you know you have it.

Natural treatments such as dietary changes, proper supplementation, exercise, detoxing (if needed), reducing stress, and other things are highly effective at reversing early Hashimoto's.

Stage 2 - Subclinical Hypothyroidism (Positive Antibodies, Normal TSH)

In stage 2, the antibody infiltration of the thyroid continues to the point that normal thyroid production becomes affected.

The pituitary gland responds by increasing TSH release in an attempt to stimulate the thyroid gland to produce more thyroid hormone.

The elevation of TSH and thyroid antibody levels can be detected in lab work.

Symptoms of low thyroid may start developing, such as mild weight gain, fatigue, constipation, and even some mild hair loss. The symptoms are usually bad enough for patients to talk to their medical provider about it.

Typically, the TSH may be mildly elevated but not high enough for the provider to prescribe medication. Even if they check thyroid antibody levels, they may not be elevated enough for treatment to be recommended. In reality, this is the perfect time to start thyroid medications.

The early use of thyroid medication may help drive down thyroid antibodies and stop (or at least slow) the progression of thyroid gland damage.

Continuing the natural therapies we mentioned in Stage 1 is also crucial.

Stage 2.5 - Thyroid Hormone Fluctuation

Not every single Hashimoto's patient will go through this stage.

As I have discussed, Hashimoto's typically leads to a gradual destruction of the thyroid gland and the development of hypothyroidism.

For up to 10-20% of patients, they can also experience episodes of hyperthyroidism (high thyroid). During this stage, their thyroid may swing from hyperthyroidism to hypothyroidism and back, which can make diagnosis difficult.

For example, one month, you could experience fatigue, weight gain, and constipation, and then the next month, you could experience hot flashes, jitteriness, weight loss, and diarrhea.

The inflammation in the thyroid gland can cause excessive thyroid hormone release instead of less.

Eventually, the damage to the thyroid will result in hypothyroidism, but it is important to know that some people may experience the fluctuations we described.

Of note, Hashimoto's patients can have what we call flare-ups. During these times, the inflammation in the thyroid gland increases, typically resulting in worsening symptoms. Sometimes, a flare-up can cause hyperthyroid symptoms, while other times, it can cause symptoms of hypothyroidism.

Stage 3 - Overt Hypothyroidism (Positive Antibodies, Elevated TSH, Decreased Free T3/Free T4)

All previous stages of Hashimoto's will end up here without treatment.

In this stage, the autoimmune damage to the thyroid has reached the point that it can no longer produce adequate amounts of thyroid hormone.

Not only are the antibody and TSH levels elevated, but now the free T3 and free T4 levels become low.

Unfortunately, this is the stage when most Hashimoto's patients are finally diagnosed. Around ten or more years have likely passed from Stage 1 to Stage 3. Thyroid medication is a necessity at this point.

Symptoms in this stage include significant weight gain, constipation, fatigue, hair loss, brittle nails, etc.

Natural therapies are still effective in Stage 3 but will require more diligence in maintaining them.

Instead of mostly avoiding gluten and dairy, a strict gluten-free, dairy-free, soy-free, or even more strict diet may be required.

Stage 4 – Additional Autoimmune Diseases

The immune dysfunction that led to the development of Hashimoto's can lead to other autoimmune conditions developing in other tissues.

If your body creates antibodies to gluten, then celiac disease develops.

If your body creates antibodies to components of your joints, then rheumatoid arthritis develops.

If your body creates antibodies to your salivary glands, then Sjogren's syndrome develops. If your body creates antibodies to your skin, then psoriasis develops.

And so on.

It is important to realize that simply treating your hypothyroidism with thyroid medication will not stop the progression of your auto-immune disease.

Be aware that other autoimmune diseases can occur in earlier stages in some people.

The point is that natural treatments and lifestyle changes are just as important as thyroid medication if you want to decrease your chances of developing other autoimmune conditions.

Stage 5 – End-stage Hashimoto's (Decreased or Negative Thyroid Antibodies)

When the thyroid antibodies continue to damage the thyroid gland for years and years, eventually, the thyroid will atrophy and basically become a lump of scar tissue. It becomes so damaged that it can no longer produce thyroid hormone and is effectively dead.

Those patients are in the same position as someone who has had their thyroid removed or destroyed by radioactive iodine. Without any thyroid production, these patients will need thyroid hormone for the rest of their lives. Without it, they would eventually die.

In addition, by the time someone gets to this stage, it is common to find that their thyroid antibody levels begin to decline and may even drop to zero.

This level is typically reached after someone has had Hashimoto's for 20 or 30 years. Preventative therapies are not going to help at this point.

However, optimizing thyroid medication, supplements, and lifestyle changes is still critical to get people feeling as good as they can.

SYMPTOMS OF HASHIMOTO'S

I discussed many of these symptoms as they related to the particular stages of Hashimoto's. For completeness and reference, I will list them again here.

EARLY HASHIMOTO'S SYMPTOMS

- Mild fatigue
- 5- 10-pound weight gain
- Depressed mood
- Difficulty focusing
- Dry skin, dry and brittle hair, nonspecific rashes
- Mild constipation
- Mild fluid retention (especially in the face and lower extremities)
- Voice changes or the sensation of throat swelling
- Reduced ability to sweat
- Mild joint pain and muscle aches
- Mild to moderate changes in the menstrual cycle

HYPERTHYROID SYMPTOMS

- Hot flashes or episodes of heat intolerance
- Jitteriness
- Anxiety
- Fatigue or big swings in energy level
- Insomnia
- Facial flushing
- Heart palpitations or racing pulse
- Weight loss or weight gain

ADVANCED HASHIMOTO'S SYMPTOMS

- Extreme fatigue/exhaustion
- Moderate weight gain (usually 20-30 pounds)
- Hair loss or hair thinning
- Mood changes, typically depression
- Menstrual irregularities
- Chronic and debilitating muscle or joint pain
- Chronic constipation, other GI issues such as gas/bloating, SIBO, acid reflux, low stomach acid

HOW TO DIAGNOSE HASHIMOTO'S

Hashimoto's can be diagnosed in three different ways:

- Positive thyroid antibodies
- Positive thyroid ultrasound
- Positive thyroid biopsy (fine needle aspiration)

Hashimoto's has a distinctive look on ultrasound that radiologists can identify. Although most patients will never need a thyroid biopsy, Hashimoto's can also be definitively identified microscopically by a trained pathologist.

By far, the most common way to diagnose Hashimoto's is by checking thyroid antibody levels.

Several steps should be considered to help diagnose Hashimoto's and fully evaluate its effect on your body:

1. Get a Complete Thyroid Panel

Hashimoto's cannot be diagnosed with just TSH or thyroid hormone levels.

The two thyroid antibodies used to diagnose Hashimoto's are thyroid peroxidase (TPO) antibodies and thyroglobulin antibodies.

If either the TPO or thyroglobulin antibodies are **greater than 35 ng/mL**, the diagnosis of Hashimoto's can be made.

Statistically, 90% of Hashimoto's patients have elevated TPO antibodies, and 80% have elevated thyroglobulin antibodies.

Keep in mind that end-stage (Stage 5) Hashimoto's patients may actually have normal thyroid antibody levels. By that time, essentially all of the thyroid gland has been destroyed, so our immune system has no need to continue to make antibodies against an "enemy" that is already dead.

2. Consider Getting a Thyroid Ultrasound

It is generally recommended that all patients diagnosed with Hashimoto's should have a thyroid ultrasound to rule out thyroid cancer.

If the ultrasound is normal, it should be repeated every two years.

If the ultrasound shows an enlarging thyroid, a repeat ultrasound should be performed every six months.

3. Evaluate for Inflammation

It is also a good idea to monitor the level of inflammation in your body if you have Hashimoto's.

Inflammation itself can worsen thyroid function by reducing T4 to T3 conversion.[15] It can also worsen insulin resistance and adrenal dysfunction.[16]

All these issues can lead to worsening fatigue, weight gain, and other symptoms that can worsen the hypothyroid symptoms that are already present.

Inflammation can be evaluated by checking an erythrocyte sedimentation rate (ESR), C-reactive protein (CRP), and ferritin levels.

If any or all of these tests are elevated, it is a sign that significant inflammation is occurring in your body and should be further evaluated.

4. Look for Other Autoimmune Conditions

Up to 5% of Hashimoto's patients have celiac disease. Inversely, up to 50% of celiac patients have Hashimoto's.[17] It is therefore recommended that all patients diagnosed with Hashimoto's should be tested for celiac disease.

Other autoimmune disorders should also be considered and tested for if you have any symptoms that could be suggestive of them. These include things such as Type 1 diabetes, psoriasis, rheumatoid arthritis, multiple sclerosis, lupus, and others.

5. Consider Testing for Hashimoto's if You Have a Mood Disorder

Studies have shown a link between depression, anxiety, and other mood disorders with Hashimoto's.[18]

If you suffer from any type of mood disorder, consider getting a complete thyroid panel lab work.

Instead of taking antidepressants or anti-anxiety medications, you may need your Hashimoto's treated primarily.

TREATMENTS FOR HASHIMOTO'S

There are two main groups of thought when it comes to treating Hashimoto's thyroiditis.

- The conventional approach
- The alternative approach

Understanding both of these approaches will help you determine which one you want to consider for your individual case.

The **conventional approach** is basically a "wait-and-see approach." It looks exactly how it sounds.[19] In this approach, your medical provider may identify the presence of thyroid antibodies and diagnose you with Hashimoto's. From that point forward, they will check your TSH and possibly T4 levels periodically until eventually they become abnormal.

Once your TSH level becomes elevated, the medical provider will start you on levothyroxine or Synthroid, which you will be on for the rest of your life. This treatment logic stems from the fact that autoimmune diseases are notoriously difficult to treat, and there are no FDA-approved medication options for treating Hashimoto's.

Instead, the idea is to wait until some or all of the thyroid gland is destroyed to the point that thyroid medication is required.

In the **alternative approach**, the medical provider attempts to use various therapies such as diet, stress reduction, exercise, toxin reduction, target supplements, and other interventions in an attempt to normalize immune function and reduce the autoimmune attack on the body.

So, which approach is better?

That really depends on what you are looking for.

If you want the simplest and least invasive therapy for your current lifestyle, then the conventional approach may be best for you.

If you want to at least try to slow down or reverse the autoimmune issue that is the root issue with Hashimoto's, then the alternative approach may be your best choice.

I was a conventional family medicine doctor for almost 22 years. I then transitioned into a functional medicine doctor, so I am obviously biased toward identifying the root issues and correcting them when possible.

Keep in mind that Hashimoto's is not benign. In addition to the hypothyroidism that it causes, there are other potential consequences that can occur in the body.

The presence of anti-TPO antibodies can be used as a long-term predictor of health in older women and may increase the risk of developing certain cancers such as breast cancer and colon cancer.[20]

Although they aren't easy, the lifestyle changes and other aspects of the alternative approach are not dangerous and at least give you a chance at slowing or reversing the autoimmune damage that is occurring in your thyroid gland.

Just be aware that not all alternative therapies are deeply tested, and they may not work consistently for each patient.

For example, diets such as the Autoimmune Protocol (AIP) diet have been used effectively to treat other autoimmune diseases such as inflammatory bowel disease (IBD).[21] Even though there may not be definitive data on using it to treat Hashimoto's, it makes intuitive sense that it could have similar benefits in Hashimoto's that it has for IBD.

If you decide to try the alternative approach, you will probably need to seek out physicians who specialize in integrative, functional, or holistic medicine. This often means they will not participate in the insurance model of medical care.

ALTERNATIVE TREATMENT APPROACH FOR HASHIMOTO'S THYROIDITIS

- Diet
- Supplements
- Treat any chronic infections
- Evaluate and treat gut dysbiosis/dysfunction
- Consider LDN
- Stress Reduction
- NDT medication
- Testosterone therapy if testosterone deficient

ALTERNATIVE MEDICINE TREATMENT APPROACH TO HASHIMOTO'S

1. Diet

Diet is one of the best ways to address immune function and treat Hashimoto's.

While there aren't many studies that have shown one particular diet is more effective than others at reducing autoimmunity, many of my patients have had significant success with certain diets for their Hashimoto's.

Because of the link between gluten sensitivity and autoimmune diseases, many providers recommend a gluten-free diet. Many patients also benefit from removing dairy from their diet.

A 2015 survey of 2,232 patients with Hashimoto's asked patients how they felt after being on a gluten-free diet and on a dairy-free diet. The results were interesting:

Gluten-free diet
- 88% felt better
- 0.73% felt worse
- 33% had reduced thyroid antibodies

Dairy-free diet
- 79% felt better
- 1.5% felt worse
- 20% had reduced thyroid antibodies

Another study showed that 76 percent of people with Hashimoto's in the study tested positive for lactose intolerance. Their TSH levels dropped significantly after going on a lactose-free diet, and they absorbed their thyroid medication more effectively.[22]

Other diets that I have found to be effective for Hashimoto's are the AIP diet, the ketogenic diet, the carnivore diet, the Paleo diet, and Whole 30.

Any diet that removes highly processed foods, gluten, sugar, and dairy may reduce your symptoms and help low antibody levels.

Keep in mind that a diet that worked for a friend or even a relative may not work for you. Diets should be personalized. You may need to try several before you find the one that works best for you.

2. Supplements for Hashimoto's

A book on this subject alone could easily be written. The information is extensive and sometimes confusing.

To make matters even worse, there aren't good ways to test the levels of many nutrients these supplements replace.

Many will require a trial-and-error approach. If you feel better or your thyroid function improves when taking one of them, you are likely deficient, and taking the supplement is important. If you notice no improvement, your time and money would likely best be served in other treatment options.

Zinc – Zinc is extremely important for patients with Hashimoto's. It plays a role in regulating the immune system as well as thyroid function.

In addition, we know that many patients with Hashimoto's are zinc deficient.

Zinc helps Hashimoto's patients by improving T4 to T3 conversion, reducing inflammation[23], boosting and regulating immune function[24], and helping with hair growth.

The best forms of zinc are zinc chelate, zinc monomethionine, zinc gluconate, zinc acetate, and zinc citrate.

Recommended dosage is 5-15 mg daily. Higher doses can cause GI upset.

Selenium – Selenium is essential for the production of the powerful antioxidant glutathione. Glutathione helps protect the thyroid gland from inflammation and free radical damage.

In addition, selenium also helps with T4 to T3 conversion.[25]

Selenium has even been shown to help reduce thyroid antibody levels in some people.[26]

Recommended forms of selenium include selenomethionine, selenocysteine, and selenium glycinate.

Normal dosage is 100-200 mcg daily.

Adrenal Support – In my experience, essentially every thyroid patient has some level of adrenal problems. Even small changes in cortisol levels can impact TSH levels and thyroid function.[27]

Stress for a prolonged period of time puts a strain on the adrenal system. As its function wanes, it can also put negative pressure on the thyroid system.

Supporting the adrenal system with quality supplements can substantially improve symptoms such as severe fatigue, "wired but tired" sensation, insomnia, and people who have mid-afternoon energy crashes.

Adrenal supplements come in the form of adrenal glandulars and adrenal adaptogens.

Glandulars contain parts of animal adrenal glands that have been dried and ground into powder form.

Adaptogens are plant-based herbs that have been shown to boost thyroid function and improve the body's ability to tolerate stress. Of the adaptogens, I have found the most effective to be ashwagandha, ifidoba, and Maca root, although there are several others that can be beneficial.

Typically, both adrenal glandulars and adaptogens may be needed if a patient is having severe symptoms. Once they start improving, it may be possible to stop the glandulars and only take adaptogens.

Probiotics and Prebiotics – I list these because the gut is a major site of immune regulation. Improving gut function can help increase T3 levels.

Probiotics act to help repopulate your gut with healthy bacteria, improve bacterial diversity, fight pathogens, reduce gut inflammation, and encourage the growth of healthy bacteria.

There isn't one "best" probiotic that patients with Hashimoto's should take. Instead, you should focus on taking probiotics that have a wide diversity of bacterial species and that have a high enough dose to have an impact.

Probiotics that we have successfully used include those with lacto-bacillus, ifidobacterium, saccharomyces boulardii, spore-based, and soil-based probiotics.

Vitamin D3 – Vitamin D is crucial for many systems in the body, including the thyroid.

Normal thyroid function is critical to achieving and maintaining normal vitamin D levels.

Low thyroid impairs intestinal absorption of vitamin D and normal activation of vitamin D.

Conversely, low vitamin D impairs T4 to T3 conversion and suppresses thyroid hormone levels.[28]

Vitamin D deficiency may also increase your risk of developing thyroid cancer.[29]

Vitamin D levels can be checked by getting a 25-OH-vitamin D blood level. Optimal levels are 50-80 ng/mL.

Most people will need a dose of vitamin D3 in the 3000-10,000IU daily range to maintain optimal blood levels. If you work indoors and have limited sunlight exposure, or if it is wintertime, higher doses may be needed to maintain optimal levels.

As a general rule, I recommend vitamin D3 in combination with vitamin K2, which helps with calcium processing, although some patients may not need the K2.

Fish Oil – Fish oil is an ideal supplement for Hashimoto's because it targets several areas that can be a problem for Hashimoto's patients. These include inflammation, immune dysregulation, mood disorders, insulin resistance, dry skin, and weight loss resistance.

It is important to buy only high-quality fish oil supplements. iFOS 5-star certified products are the best. A combination of both EPA and DHA in the 1000-2000 mg dose is also ideal. During a Hashimoto's flare-up, taking 2000-4000 mg daily may be helpful.

Glutathione – In a healthy body with normal thyroid function, glutathione is produced to clean up free radicals produced with the creation of thyroid hormone.

When the thyroid is dysfunctional, such as in Hashimoto's, glutathione production decreases, which results in an increase of free radicals that damage the thyroid gland.

Since selenium is necessary for normal glutathione production, selenium supplements (which I discussed earlier) are very beneficial.

Oral glutathione is also available and has been shown to be safe in dosages from 250-1000 mg daily, although much lower dosages may still be helpful in Hashimoto's.

Iodine - If you or someone you know has had Hashimoto's for any length of time, you have likely heard or read about the controversy of iodine supplementation.

It is important to remember that iodine is an element that is necessary for life.

Thyroid cells are the only cells in the body that can absorb iodine. Thyroid cells then combine iodine with tyrosine to make thyroid hormone.

Without iodine, there would be no thyroid hormone production. Without thyroid hormones, life is not possible.

Studies have indeed shown that iodine in high doses can increase thyroid antibody levels. That fact has been borne out by the skyrocketing levels of thyroid disease since developed countries began adding iodine to their water supplies. However, we believe that most people who react negatively to iodine lack other nutrients and antioxidants, such as selenium, which are required to reduce thyroid gland damage when thyroid hormone is created.

Most of the needed daily iodine can be obtained from eating foods such as bananas, strawberries, milk, yogurt, and eggs.

For those patients who need more, I recommend using a lower dose combined with zinc, selenium, glutathione, and other antioxidants.

3. Low-Dose Naltrexone (LDN)

This medication may surprise you by being listed here. LDN is an opioid antagonist, which means it blocks opioid receptors in the brain.

When taken in doses of 50-100 mg, it completely saturates the opioid receptors, which prevents the "high" that would normally be experienced from taking narcotic medications. It is, therefore, used by people in drug or alcohol rehab to help them stay off their drug abuse.

When taken in very low doses (1.5 mg-6 mg typically), LDN increases the level of endorphins in the brain.

Endorphins appear to modulate the immune system. Therefore, raising endorphin levels impacts the immune system in a positive way.

LDN decreases inflammation in chronic pain conditions.[30] It appears to be particularly helpful in patients who have chronic pain as one of their symptoms.

The majority of research on LDN primarily focuses on other autoimmune conditions, such as multiple sclerosis (MS) and Crohn's disease, and chronic pain conditions, such as fibromyalgia.

For Hashimoto's, LDN appears to improve things by:
- Increasing conversion of T4 to T3[31]
- Increasing total T3 levels
- Reducing autoantibody levels[32]

Much of the evidence supporting the use of LDN in Hashimoto's is anecdotal, meaning doctors and patients give their personal experience using it. I personally have seen a definite improvement in many patients.

There are websites such as http://www.lowdosenaltrexone.org that will show much of the research and patient testimonials about LDN.

Another big plus for many patients regarding LDN is it can help with weight loss. It is even marketed with bupropion as a weight loss drug called Contrave.

Typical dosage is 1.5 mg at bedtime for a couple of weeks, then increased to 3 mg. You can continue to increase the dose as needed up to 6 mg.

There are two main side effects to keep in mind: It can cause vivid dreams in some people. More importantly, it can cause a major withdrawal if you are taking narcotic pain medication regularly. If that is the case, do NOT take LDN until you are off all opioids (narcotics).

4. Black Seed Oil

If you have any experience with integrative or functional medicine, then you have likely heard of black seed oil and its many benefits.

If you come from a purely conventional medicine background, you may have no idea what I'm talking about.

Black cumin (also known as Nigella sativa) is a medicinal plant that has been used for thousands of years. The oil from its seeds is used for things such as inflammation, cardiovascular health, infections, and skin issues. It is also commonly used for nausea, diarrhea, the common cold, and headaches.

The primary active ingredient in black seed oil is thymoquinone.

There are studies using black seed oil in the treatment of Hashimoto's.

A 2016 study from Iran showed a reduction in weight plus weight and hip circumference. TSH levels also significantly dropped, and serum T3 levels increased. TPO antibody levels were also slightly reduced.[37]

Another study showed that black seed oil significantly reduced body weight and BMI. LDL cholesterol and triglycerides also decreased, while HDL levels increased. All participants in the study had Hashimoto's.[38]

Typical dose is 1-2 grams daily. It comes in capsule, powder, or liquid forms.

5. Stress Reduction

Although I have discussed this topic in other chapters, it is important to mention it again here.

Stress is a major source of inflammation in the body. This can come in the form of physical, mental, and emotional.

There is good evidence that certain therapies, such as mindfulness and meditation, reduce markers of inflammation, improve cell-mediated immunity, and decrease biological aging. (33)

Obviously, reducing or eliminating any sources of stress in your life will be invaluable. Learning to better manage the stress you can't remove or reduce can be just as important. This may improve your immune function, which can reduce your autoimmunity.

6. Treat Any Chronic Infections

Patients with a chronic infection, such as EBV, CMV, or others, may benefit from antiviral supplements and/or medications. There is very little in the way of clinical studies to support this, but there is substantial anecdotal evidence showing it can be beneficial for some patients.

7. Evaluate Gut Function

Because the gut plays a central role in immunity and gut dysfunction may lead to intestinal permeability (leaky gut), targeting it for improvement is a logical goal.

Addressing digestive issues such as acid reflux, SIBO, leaky gut, and dysbiosis may help impact immune function and decrease autoantibody levels.[34]

8. Thyroid Medications

The alternative medicine treatment approach for Hashimoto's typically uses different thyroid medication than the conventional approach.

NDT thyroid medications such as Armour Thyroid, Naturethroid, and NP Thyroid contain both T4 and T3.

Some studies and surveys suggest that Hashimoto's patients respond better and feel better using these medications over levothyroxine.

There is one thing to keep in mind. Since NDT is derived from porcine (pig), people may be sensitive to them or even trigger auto-immunity from using them. That is extremely rare in my experience, but something to keep in mind.

9. Testosterone Therapy

Hopefully, at this point in the book, I have adequately shown that the hormonal systems in the body interact with each other and are dependent on each other for optimal function.

We know from several studies that optimizing thyroid function can boost testosterone and estrogen production. There is even evidence that testosterone therapy in men can reduce thyroid antibody levels in patients with Hashimoto's.[35]

If you are diagnosed with low testosterone, testosterone replacement therapy could have a positive impact on your Hashimoto's.

PROGNOSIS

If you have Hashimoto's thyroiditis and no treatments are given or lifestyle changes made, you will eventually develop hypothyroidism.

That is the primary stance regarding Hashimoto's in conventional medicine. And if nothing is done, that is exactly what will happen.

Just like with any other autoimmune condition, however, it is possible for Hashimoto's to spontaneously resolve on its own. One study showed spontaneous recovery can happen in over 20% of cases.[36] I believe that number can be even higher when Hashimoto's is caught in its early stages and appropriate treatments are begun.

Permanent hypothyroidism doesn't have to be the inevitable result of Hashimoto's.

SUMMARY

- Hashimoto's is the most common autoimmune condition in the world, affecting up to 10% of the US adult population.

- The cause of Hashimoto's is not exactly known, but it appears to require a genetic predisposition that is then activated by some type of trigger.

- Triggers can include stress, infections such as EBV and H. pylori, nutrient deficiencies, gut dysbiosis/dysfunction, and food sensitivities/allergies.

- Diagnosis of Hashimoto's includes checking lab tests for two different thyroid antibodies: TPO antibodies and thyroglobulin antibodies.

- Thyroid ultrasound is recommended at initial diagnosis and every two years afterward. If it is growing, then the ultrasound should be repeated every six months.

- It is important to evaluate for inflammation and other autoimmune diseases if you have Hashimoto's.

- Consider testing for Hashimoto's if you have a mood disorder, such as anxiety, depression, or bipolar disorder.

- There are several stages of Hashimoto's that differ based on how long the patient has had the condition and the presence and level of thyroid antibodies and hypothyroidism.

- Conventional treatment for Hashimoto's typically consists of a "wait-and-see" approach. This consists of monitoring the TSH periodically and starting levothyroxine if needed.

- Alternative treatment for Hashimoto's includes diet, targeted supplements, stress reduction, treating chronic infections such as EBV, evaluating gut function, NDT thyroid medication, and low-dose naltrexone. Testosterone therapy can be beneficial if you also have testosterone deficiency.

- 20% of patients with Hashimoto's may spontaneously recover. The other 80% will eventually develop hypothyroidism if no lifestyle or other treatments are initiated early.

6.

HYPERTHYROIDISM AND GRAVE'S DISEASE

Albert is a 68-year-old Chinese American male who came to the office for Graves' disease management. He had seen a local endocrinologist who recommended radioactive iodine ablation (RAI) for his condition. Albert wanted to see if there were any therapies besides RAI that might help him.

He was diagnosed about three months prior to his appointment with me. He had an extremely stressful job, and his wife died after a long battle with cancer in the past year. He was started on a beta-blocker to control his heart rate. He had lost around 30 pounds in those six months, felt constantly anxious and jittery, had frequent diarrhea, and had a tremor when he tried to do tasks such as writing his name.

Lab testing showed a TSH of <0.005, a free T4 of 4.2 pmol/L, free T3 of 8.6 pmol/L, thyroglobulin ab of 424 IU/mL, and a TSI index of 2.73 (273%).

His blood pressure was 108/62, pulse was 114, and temperature was 99.1°.

He was diagnosed with Graves' disease and Hashimoto's. He was placed on a whole-food, gluten-free, dairy-free diet. He was prescribed methimazole 5 mg three times daily. The beta-blocker was continued. He also started selenium 200 mcg daily, zinc 30 mg daily, vitamin D3 5000u daily, and fish oil 1000 mg twice daily. He was encouraged to see a counselor to deal with the death of his wife.

Albert came back to the clinic two months later and stated he felt much better. His weight loss had stopped, as had his tremors and feelings of anxiety. He was seeing his counselor on a regular basis, which seemed to be helping with his grief. He was mostly following a gluten-free diet.

He followed a few months later and was still feeling well. No hypothyroid symptoms.

Lab work on the follow-up visit showed a TSH of 1.258, free T4 of 1.33, free T3 of 3.1, and a TSI index of 2.57 (257%).

CAUSES OF HYPERTHYROIDISM

Hyperthyroidism occurs when an excessive amount of thyroid hormone is present in the body. It occurs in 0.8% of the US population and 1.3% in Europe. It is five times more common in women than in men. In older women, the prevalence increases to 4 or 5%.

Hyperthyroidism can be caused by several conditions:

1. Graves' Disease - This will be discussed in detail later in this chapter.

2. Toxic Nodule or Toxic Nodular Goiter - Refers to one or more nodules (typically benign) that develop in the thyroid gland.

The nodules produce excessive amounts of thyroid hormone and do not respond to the normal TSH signaling from the pituitary gland.

They are called "toxic" due to the hyperthyroid symptoms that result from the high thyroid hormone levels.

Keep in mind that if there is more than one nodule, not all the nodules may be over-producing thyroid hormone.

The nodules may or may not be palpable on a physical exam.

Typically, the nodules can be identified either through a thyroid ultrasound or via a radioactive iodine uptake scan. That is why all new cases of hyperthyroidism should have a thyroid ultrasound to help identify the cause.

3. Thyroiditis - Hashimoto's, Postpartum

By this point in the book, you hopefully have a fairly comfortable grasp of Hashimoto's.

While Hashimoto's classically causes hypothyroidism, it can periodically have flare-ups when the inflammation within the thyroid gland causes excess thyroid hormone to be released.

This is especially true in the early stages of Hashimoto's. I call it stage 2.5.

The diagnosis can be confirmed by checking TPO antibodies, thyroglobulin antibodies, and thyroid-stimulating immunoglobulins (TSI). If TPO antibodies and/or thyroglobulin antibodies are positive, but TSI is negative, then the hyperthyroidism is probably due to Hashimoto's and not Graves'.

Postpartum thyroiditis is an autoimmune disease very similar to Hashimoto's. It occurs in the first year after delivery in women with no prior history of thyroid disease.[1]

It can lead to transient or permanent thyroid disease.

32% of patients have transient hyperthyroidism, 43% have transient hypothyroidism, and 25% have transient hyperthyroidism that eventually converts to hypothyroidism.

The TPO antibodies are typically elevated in postpartum thyroiditis.

Most cases will return to normal thyroid function within 12-18 months.

4. Pituitary Tumors

Benign growths in the pituitary gland (called adenomas) are a rare cause of hyperthyroidism.

Typically, the tumors suppress TSH release from the pituitary, which results in decreased thyroid hormone production and subsequent hypothyroidism.

However, in 1% of cases, the pituitary adenoma can secrete excessive amounts of TSH.
(2) This results in overproduction of thyroid hormone by the thyroid gland and hyperthyroidism.

Of note, there are even rare cases of patients with both Graves' disease and a TSH-secreting pituitary adenoma.[3]

If someone is getting treated for Graves' disease but continues to have hyperthyroid labs and symptoms, an MRI of the pituitary may be needed to assess for any adenomas.

5. Thyroid Cancer

Thyroid cancers may sometimes result in the excessive production of thyroid hormones. Conversely, hyperthyroidism itself increases the risk of thyroid cancer developing.

That makes sense if you think about it.

When there is hyperthyroidism, there is increased activity in the thyroid gland, which causes the increased amount of thyroid hormone in the body. Anytime there is an increase in cellular activity, the odds are increased that some cells may be produced that are abnormal (cancerous).

Some studies have even shown that thyroid-stimulating antibodies that are present in Graves' disease may promote tumor growth by activating TSH receptors in thyroid cancer cells.[4]

Again, it is important that hyperthyroid patients have a thyroid ultrasound. If the ultrasound shows one or more nodules, then a radioactive iodine uptake and scan or FNA (fine needle aspiration) should be performed to rule in or out the possibility of any malignancy.

6. Excessive Thyroid Medication

I actually see this fairly often.

Many people get frustrated because they are convinced they have a thyroid issue, but their medical provider either disagrees or only puts them on a low dose of levothyroxine, which doesn't relieve their symptoms.

So, out of desperation, they buy one of the over-the-counter thyroid glandular products.

With limited dosage options and little to no regulation of these products, they end up taking way more thyroid hormone than is needed, which puts them in a hyperthyroid state.

Another possibility is someone has unknowingly had remission of their Hashimoto's or hypothyroidism, but they continue to take their regular dose of thyroid medication, which makes them hyperthyroid.

And yet another scenario is someone being treated for hypothyroidism but isn't feeling any better. They then increase their dose on their own, which pushes them into hyperthyroidism.

Getting a full thyroid history, which includes medications, their dosages, and a complete supplement list, is critical to help identify the cause of hyperthyroidism.

GRAVES' DISEASE

Graves' disease is the most common cause of hyperthyroidism.

The term Graves' disease pays homage to Irish physician Robert Graves. In 1835, he published lectures describing several cases of cardiac palpitations associated with enlargement of the thyroid gland and bulging eyes (exophthalmos) in one case.

Other people had actually described similar cases years or even centuries before Graves, but his name has been forever linked to the condition.

Graves' disease is an autoimmune disease that results in an overactive thyroid (hyperthyroidism). It is also known as diffuse toxic hyperplasia or diffuse toxic goiter.

The immune system begins attacking the thyroid gland, which causes it to produce extra thyroid hormone.

Untreated, hyperthyroidism will cause multiple symptoms, which I will discuss later in this chapter.

We tend to think of Graves' disease as a thyroid disease. However, it's really more of a disease of the immune system.[5] If you can manage your immune system, you can reduce the impact and damage that it is causing to your thyroid gland.

Just like with Hashimoto's, we don't know exactly what causes Graves' disease. There seems to be a genetic predisposition that is activated by some type of trigger.

COMMON GRAVES' DISEASES TRIGGERS

- Infections – EBV, bacterial
- Gut dysbiosis
- Environmental toxins – heavy metals, ect
- Dietary issues – gluten, ect
- Excessive iodine intake
- Stress – physical and emotional

Examples of these triggers include:

Infections, particularly viral or bacterial[6] - Just like Hashimoto's, Graves' disease appears to have a strong link to infections such as EBV virus and others.

EBV is very effective at evading our immune system and setting up house somewhere in our body.

Over 90% of the world's population has been exposed to EBV.

Most people are able to get the infection under control, but a percentage of them develop a chronic EBV infection that triggers an abnormal immune response that can lead to autoantibodies being developed against parts of the body, including the thyroid gland.

A similar story can be told about helicobacter pylori infections of the gut. Low stomach acid creates an environment where H. pylori can thrive. H. pylori infections can trigger autoimmune reactions such as Hashimoto's or Graves' disease.

Fortunately, it can be eradicated with multiple antibiotics and other medications, so testing for it if you have any GI symptoms (acid reflux, dysbiosis, etc.) can be beneficial.

Gut dysbiosis and/or inflammation - Since the gut is a major player in our immune system, it makes sense that any dysfunction could affect our immune system.

If the delicate balance of healthy bacteria in our gut (called the microbiome) gets out of balance for any reason (stress, poor diet, frequent antibiotics, acid-blocking drugs, etc.), it can create an environment where opportunistic bacteria or fungi can overgrow in the gut.

Improving gut dysbiosis likely won't cure Graves' disease, but it will help reduce symptoms and other complications by maximizing the immune response in the body.

Environmental toxins such as chemicals and heavy metals[7]
Exposure to environmental toxins such as lead, mercury, and aluminum has been shown to increase the risk of autoantibody production, including thyroid autoantibodies.

Dietary - Gluten and dairy intolerance/sensitivity are finally being recognized as common and dangerous conditions.

Consuming these products if you have an intolerance leads to an increase in inflammation in the lining of the gut, which results in intestinal permeability (leaky gut). This allows foreign bacteria to enter the bloodstream that normally would not.

These unwelcome visitors trigger a strong immune response, which can lead to autoantibody production and the development of an autoimmune condition.

Excessive iodine exposure - Excessive iodine exposure from drugs (such as amiodarone), food preservatives, large fish, and other sources have been shown to trigger hyperthyroidism and Graves'.[8]

Stress (physical and emotional) - Stress is quite possibly the number one trigger for thyroid autoimmune disease (Hashimoto's and Graves').

The physical or emotional stress likely activates the genetic predisposition, which results in autoantibody production.

There are likely many other potential triggers, but these are the most common in my experience. If possible, it is always beneficial to try to find out what may have triggered your Graves' disease. Treating that cause has the potential to improve or even reverse the disease.

Much of this chapter will sound like a repeat of the Hashimoto's chapter. There is a good reason for that. The two conditions are similar in that they both are the result of autoantibodies that attack the thyroid gland.

Graves' disease results in increased thyroid hormone levels, while Hashimoto's typically results in decreased thyroid hormone levels.

As I discussed, however, sometimes Hashimoto's can cause episodes of hyperthyroidism, which can make the diagnosis confusing and difficult at times.

It is even possible to have BOTH Graves' disease and Hashimoto's, which is another reason it is important to get antibody levels checked to help you make the best treatment decisions.

SYMPTOMS

Because Graves' disease impacts your thyroid, it can and will cause a diverse set of symptoms.

Your thyroid helps to manage and even control almost every system in the body. This includes things such as other hormones, hair and nail growth, weight, GI function, and more.

So, it should come as no surprise that Graves' disease can cause a wide array of symptoms from various systems of your body. The resulting hyperthyroidism has the effect of activating all of these other systems.

What does that mean exactly?

For example, since your thyroid helps to control your weight, increasing thyroid hormone levels will increase your metabolism and result in weight loss.[9]

If you apply the same logic to other bodily systems, you can intuitively compile this list of common Graves' disease symptoms:

GRAVES'S DISEASES COMMON SYMPTOMS

- Hair loss (Dry & brittle hair)
- Diarrhea or increased BM's
- Tremors or shaking hands
- Anxiety or racing thoughts
- Rapid heart rate
- Chest pain
- Shortness of breath
- Weight loss
- Changes in menstrual cycle
- Infertility
- Heat sensitivity
- Decreased energy
- Insomnia or restless sleep
- Bulging eyes

All these symptoms are the result of overactivation of the various body systems due to an excess of thyroid hormone.

The good news is that almost all the symptoms can be managed by getting thyroid function into the optimal range.

Long-term Graves' disease can lead to several dangerous conditions. The two most common that we want to prevent are atrial fibrillation and osteoporosis.[10, 11]

DIAGNOSIS

Compared to other thyroid diseases, it is pretty easy to diagnose Graves' disease. There are three main ways to diagnose Graves' disease:

1. Thyroid Lab Tests

This is typically the first step taken to diagnose Graves' disease.

The TSH is typically suppressed (close to 0) or very low, the free T3 and free T4 levels are high, and one or more thyroid antibodies are high.

The primary thyroid antibody that we check for Graves' disease is called the thyroid stimulating immunoglobulin (TSI).[12]

A positive TSI antibody level is highly predictive of Graves'.[13]

The standard range for TSI is measured as a percentage. Any level greater than 1.4 (140%) is highly predictable for Graves'. Any level that is nearing 1.3 to 1.4 should be monitored regularly because that person is likely to develop Graves' in the near future.

Extremely high levels of thyroid hormone (free T4 and free T3) may result in severe symptoms, or a condition known as a **thyroid storm**, which is a medical emergency.[14] In that situation, medical care should be pursued immediately because hospitalization may be required.

2. Thyroid Ultrasound

A thyroid ultrasound should be performed on any person with hyperthyroidism.

Even though Graves' disease is the most common cause, there are other potential causes that should be ruled out, such as toxic nodules or even thyroid cancer.

Typically, Graves' disease will result in either a normal-appearing thyroid gland or a diffusely enlarged gland without nodules (called a goiter).

If one or more nodules are found on thyroid ultrasound, a radioactive iodine uptake and scan should be performed.

3. Radioactive Iodine Uptake (RAIU) and Scan Test

This test measures how much radioactive iodine is absorbed by the thyroid gland, using a controlled amount of radioactive iodine in a specific timeframe.

During the test, a pre-measured amount of radioactive iodine is swallowed up to 24 hours before the test.

The level of radioactivity in the thyroid gland is then measured at certain intervals hours later using a device called a gamma probe, which is placed over the front of the neck.

The original amount of thyroid hormone, which was measured in the blood before the tests, is compared to the amount of radioactivity measured after taking the radioactive iodine.

The radioactive amount is listed as a percentage of the original amount.

Any 24-hour result greater than 35% is considered abnormal and needs further workup and treatment.

If there are nodules, then assessing the uptake of each nodule is important.

If the nodule is "hot," that means it has increased uptake, which is typical of a toxic nodule.

If the nodule is "cold," then a biopsy is likely indicated to rule out malignancy. Most biopsies can be performed via a fine needle aspiration either by an endocrinologist or a surgeon.

TESTING RESULTS FOUND IN GRAVES' DISEASE

- TSH – low or suppressed
- Free T4 – elevated
- Free T3 – elevated
- TSI - > 1.4 (140%)
- RAIU Scan - > 35%
- Thyroid U/S – diffuse inflammation and enlargement

TREATMENT

Treatments for Graves' disease focus on reducing or slowing down the thyroid function. As this occurs, the symptoms typically resolve rather quickly.

These treatments are typically fairly simple. However, finding the right balance of thyroid hormone can be quite a challenge.

For example, if your thyroid is producing 150% of the optimal amount of thyroid hormone that your body needs, it is very difficult to reduce thyroid hormone production to exactly 100%.

Instead, the medications, surgery, and radiation that we will be describing later often reduce thyroid hormone production to as little as 0%. So, the typical Graves' patient goes from a hyperthyroid state to a severely hypothyroid state after treatment.

Here is a list of the conventional treatments available for Graves' disease:

- **Anti-Thyroid Medication (Beta-blockers, methimazole, PTU)**

  These medications either block the **effect** of thyroid hormone or block the **production** and **conversion** of thyroid hormone.

  Beta-blockers such as propranolol help reduce the impact of excessive thyroid hormone on cardiac tissue by slowing down the heart rate and reducing the sensation of palpitations.[15]

They also help to block the effects of adrenaline, which can reduce hand tremors and feelings of anxiety.

However, they do nothing to treat the underlying problem.

Methimazole and **PTU** block the effects of hyperthyroidism by inhibiting the production and activation of thyroid hormone in your body.[16]

They block the enzyme called thyroid peroxidase, which is responsible for producing thyroid hormone. They also block the peripheral conversion of T4 to T3, resulting in less circulating and active T3 hormone available.

This is all very helpful in the short term. Long-term use, however, is more controversial.

While some studies show anti-thyroid medication has more favorable effects on mood, cognition, and heart function, other studies show they may cause weight gain and other harmful side effects, such as bone loss.[17, 18]

As I stated previously, anti-thyroid medication typically pushes a hyperthyroid patient into significant hypothyroidism. Untreated, this is as potentially dangerous long-term as hyperthyroidism.

The typical weight gain for someone taking methimazole is 12 pounds (5kg).[19]

It is possible (although difficult) to find a dose that will suppress excess thyroid hormone but will allow for some thyroid function to occur. It will require frequent communication with the medical provider managing your Graves' disease.

Ultimately, you may need to change to a more permanent treatment for your Graves' disease if other therapies do not help it go into remission.

- **Radioactive Iodine Ablation (RAIA) Therapy** -
  Radioactive iodine is consumed orally. The iodine is then absorbed by the thyroid gland.

In effect, the radiation from the radioactive iodine irradiates and destroys the thyroid gland.

The dose is calculated typically by a radiologist using what is called Marinelli's formula.[20]

Keep in mind that the thyroid doesn't die all at once. It could take months or even years for the thyroid gland to stop all hormone production.

In one study of 576 Graves' patients who were treated with RAI therapy, after one year, 17% were still hyperthyroid, 77% were hypothyroid, and 6% were euthyroid.[21]

Many of the patients needed a second or even third dose of RAI to fully ablate their thyroid glands.

After RAIA therapy, it is very important to do regular thyroid lab tests (typically monthly or bi-monthly) because once the levels start dropping, they typically drop fast and hard.

Thyroid medication may need to be started early and titrated rapidly, depending on the lab results. If this is not done, severe hypothyroid symptoms may hit, including rapid weight gain and severe fatigue.

- **Thyroidectomy** - The thyroid gland is completely removed surgically.

Just like after RAIA therapy, the thyroid hormone levels will need to be monitored frequently, and thyroid medication initiated at the first sign that the thyroid hormone levels begin dropping to minimize the "thyroid crash" that can occur once the patient becomes hypothyroid.

Keep in mind that the last two treatment options we discussed above will ultimately result in each patient becoming hypothyroid. Lifelong thyroid medication will be required, as we discuss in detail in Chapter 7.

NATURAL TREATMENTS FOR GRAVES' DISEASE

Natural treatments are not as extensively studied as the conventional therapies.

However, there are some small studies and multiple anecdotal cases that have shown reversal of Graves' and improvement of symptoms by using natural therapies.[22]

These treatments are normally harmless, so my stance is, why not at least try them?

I would suggest giving them a try before undergoing a permanent treatment such as thyroidectomy or RAI ablation.

NATURAL TREATMENTS FOR HYPERTHYROIDISM

- Diet
- Supplements
- Improve Gut Function
- Stress Reduction

DIET

Diet is probably the safest and potentially most effective natural treatment for Graves' Disease.

As I stated earlier, there are scientific studies that link the development of autoimmune disease to gut dysfunction and food intolerances such as celiac disease.[23]

The typical American diet is high in inflammatory fats, refined sugar, salt, and processed food. Simply reducing much of that "junk" will go a long way toward reducing your whole body's inflammation, which will only help any autoimmune disease, including Graves'.

If you are someone who does better with a list of "do not eat" foods, then these are great things to avoid:

- Gluten
- Dairy
- Common food allergens
- Foods high in iodine
- Caffeine
- Refined sugar
- Seed oils
- Processed food with preservatives

Foods that you should consume if you have hyperthyroidism:

- Healthy fats, oils, and nuts
- Organic fruits and vegetables
- Healthy sources of proteins such as wild-caught fish or free-range chicken and grass-fed beef
- Plant sources of protein such as buckwheat, hemp seeds, chia seeds, nutritional yeast, and other seeds
- Filtered water

Remember, if you have had RAIA therapy or a thyroidectomy, then you are (or will soon be) hypothyroid, and your dietary needs may change. In that case, I recommend moving on to Chapter 11 to get more specific dietary recommendations for hypothyroidism.

SUPPLEMENTS FOR GRAVES' DISEASE

The goal with supplements is to get your body into remission, or in other words, no signs or symptoms of Graves' disease.

While that may not be possible for a lot of patients, it can help with many others and is certainly worth trying before undergoing a permanent thyroid-destroying treatment.

1. Probiotics

Many autoimmune conditions may originate in your GI tract.

Various factors—stress, hormone imbalances, poor diet, nutrient deficiencies, etc. can damage the intestinal lining.

This lining is meant to act as a barrier that allows the absorption of good materials and prevents more sinister materials from being absorbed.

When damage to that lining occurs (what we call leaky gut), some of those sinister bacteria and/or undigested proteins can be absorbed, which triggers a strong immune reaction that can lead to an autoimmune disease developing.

Probiotics can help improve the microbiome of your GI tract and reduce the permeability of the intestinal lining. They can also help reduce inflammation.

Keep in mind that probiotics by themselves will likely not be enough to make a big difference in your thyroid condition.

For example, if an inflammatory condition such as small intestinal bacterial overgrowth (SIBO) or small intestinal fungal overgrowth (SIFO) are present, targeted treatments against those conditions will be required.

2. Zinc

Zinc has been shown to balance the immune system and is required for optimal immune function.[24]

Zinc also acts as a potent anti-inflammatory agent.[25]

Both of these functions are beneficial in someone with an autoimmune condition such as Graves' disease.

As an added bonus, zinc also helps to normalize T4 to T3 conversion, which is a common issue in all thyroid patients.[26]

3. Vitamin D3

In my opinion, almost every person alive would benefit from vitamin D3 supplementation. That is even truer for people with Graves' disease.

Low levels of vitamin D can exacerbate and even cause hyperthyroidism.

Fortunately, studies have shown that taking vitamin D3 may help to reverse Graves' disease.[27]

If you have Graves' disease, get your 25-OH-vitamin D level checked. Optimal levels are around 50-80 ng/mL.

4. Fish Oil

Fish oil is very helpful for Graves' disease because it is a potent anti-inflammatory agent.[28] It will be next to impossible to normalize thyroid function if inflammation levels are high.

An added benefit is fish oil has been shown to help with weight loss, especially when combined with exercise.

5. Magnesium

Thyroid dysregulation increases magnesium excretion from the kidneys. This means that thyroid patients are especially prone to developing magnesium deficiency.[29]

Add in the fact that magnesium is involved in proper immune function, and it's easy to see why magnesium supplementation may be helpful in Graves' disease patients.[30]

Magnesium can cause diarrhea and other GI issues (have you ever heard of Milk of Magnesia?), so using the right form of it is important.

For most patients, magnesium glycinate is well tolerated and effective. Typical dose is 250-500 mg daily, usually taken at bedtime.

6. High Dose Iodine

This supplement recommendation may seem strange since excess iodine is one of the causes of Graves' disease that we discussed earlier.

High doses of iodine, however, have been shown to reduce thyroid production and alter thyroid conversion in the peripheral cells.

This is called the Wolff-Chaikoff effect and is likely a mechanism designed to prevent excessive production of thyroid hormone following a large dose of iodine.[31]

This effect can be as potent as some of the prescription medications that are used to lower thyroid production in Graves' disease patients.

Using this technique could be used for temporary treatments for things such as flare-ups.

You may have heard of people exposed to radiation being treated with iodine pills. This is the same mechanism and concept.

Because iodine may temporarily block thyroid function, you should not consider this therapy without consulting with your medical provider.

A typical recommended dose for iodine is 150 mcg daily. In this situation, doses as high as 12.5 mg per day may be needed.

7. Adrenal Support

As I have discussed in previous chapters, adrenal function and thyroid function are intimately connected. Even small changes in cortisol production can have a significant impact on thyroid function.

This commonly results in symptoms such as fatigue or low energy.

Taking adrenal adaptogens has been shown to normalize cortisol levels, and many patients report having a decrease in symptoms while taking them.

Adrenal adaptogens also help your body tolerate stress, improve weight loss, and improve sleep patterns.[32]

These herbs should be a baseline treatment for essentially all people with thyroid issues. Common adrenal adaptogens include ashwagandha, rhodiola, maca root, and many others.

8. Selenium

One of the primary functions of selenium is to protect the thyroid gland from inflammation. That makes it an obvious choice for anyone with hyperthyroidism or Graves'.

Selenium reduces inflammation by helping your body produce glutathione, an extremely potent antioxidant.

Selenium is also a required component of other enzymes involved in the thyroid, known as selenoproteins.

There is even evidence that selenium can improve treatment outcomes in patients who are taking anti-thyroid drugs such as methimazole.

Typical doses of selenium are around 100-200 mcg daily.

9. Bugleweed (Lycopus) & Lemon Balm (Melissa officinalis)

These two supplements have specific actions that, when used correctly, may help to reduce thyroid function and thus help with hyperthyroidism.

These herbs can block TSH production and thyroid antibodies.[33] They also reduce T4 to T3 conversion in the peripheral tissues. The net effect is thyroid hormone levels fall.

Think of them as a weaker and more natural version of methimazole.

Unfortunately, the effect is not consistent in everyone. However, when they do work, they appear to work very well.

I do not recommend taking them if you are already on a drug such as methimazole. I would also strongly suggest discussing them with your medical provider before considering a trial of them.

10. Motherwort (Leonurus cardiac L.)

Motherwort has been shown to help block some of the extrathyroidal symptoms that hyperthyroid patients may experience, such as rapid heart rate and heart palpitations.

Think of it as a natural alternative to beta-blockers such as propranolol.

It is common to find motherwort in combination with bugleweed as a sort of natural treatment for hyperthyroidism instead of methimazole and propranolol.

Much like bugleweed, motherwort doesn't work in every situation and is not intended for long-term use.

Again, I don't recommend using motherwort without first discussing it with your medication provider, and don't use it in place of propranolol without involving your medical provider in the decision.

- **Improve Gut Function**

Your next step should be to improve your gut health.

Not only does your GI system take care of digestion, but it is also a huge component of your immune system.

Most thyroid patients, including those with Graves' disease, have problems with their gut. And a dysfunctional gut can even be the trigger for the development of Graves' disease.

Evaluating your gut microbiome, changing your diet, and taking certain supplements can all help improve your gut function, which will secondarily improve your autoimmune condition.

- **Reduce stress**

If you're stressed, just stop it. Remove all stress from your life. Wouldn't it be nice if it were that easy?

While it is obviously impossible to remove all stress, you can change how you respond to stress.

Stress may be the single largest factor in the development of inflammation and autoimmune diseases in the body.

All of these stress reduction techniques collectively can have a major impact on your stress levels.

Things to pursue include getting enough sleep, taking adrenal supplements, regular meditation, and yoga.

Please don't neglect this step.

OTHER THINGS TO CONSIDER TO TREAT HYPERTHYROIDISM

- **Consider LDN**

Low-dose naltrexone was originally created and used to treat alcohol dependence.[34]

LDN has been shown to have weight-lowering benefits and is beneficial in reducing inflammation.

LDN also modulates the immune system, which can make it helpful in treating autoimmune conditions such as Crohn's disease.[35]

It would be off-label use for Graves' disease, but with the potential to help and the minimal risk of side effects, LDN might be a reasonable option to try.

Typical doses are 1.5 mg at bedtime for 1-2 weeks, then increasing to 3 mg at bedtime. It can be titrated to 6 mg daily or even higher.

- **Add-back therapy**

Okay, this one may sound completely counterintuitive.

Why would you give levothyroxine to someone who already has too much thyroid hormone circulating in their body?

There is actually some emerging data that suggests it could help in certain situations.[36]

In many cases of hyperthyroidism and Graves' disease, patients are given antithyroid medication such as methimazole to block thyroid hormone production.

HYPERTHYROIDISM AND GRAVE'S DISEASE

The problem with this treatment is not that it doesn't work but that it often works too well. Many of those patients go from a state of excess thyroid to a state of too little thyroid.

The difficulty is finding just the right dose of antithyroid medication to get you back to a normal level of thyroid hormone.

Add-back therapy, sometimes referred to as "block and replace," is a treatment where the excess thyroid is blocked by the antithyroid medication while levothyroxine is taken in an attempt to get the thyroid hormone level back to a normal level.

This may not intuitively make sense until you understand that it is easier to dose anti-thyroid medication in higher doses than in lower doses.

Antithyroid medications are notoriously difficult to dose to the point where some thyroid hormone production still occurs.

Instead, they typically have a dose where there is not enough blockage of thyroid function; then, the very next dose may cause essentially complete blockage. It can be hard to find the middle ground between those two extremes.

Instead of constantly experimenting with different doses of the antithyroid medication, it might make sense to just completely block all thyroid hormone production and then replace what thyroid hormone is needed with a thyroid medication such as levothyroxine.

This would allow for this therapy to be used for a longer period of time (up to several years) instead of having to go to a permanent option such as thyroidectomy or RAIA.

This would also allow more time for the possibility of spontaneous remission to occur.[37]

THYROID EYE DISEASE

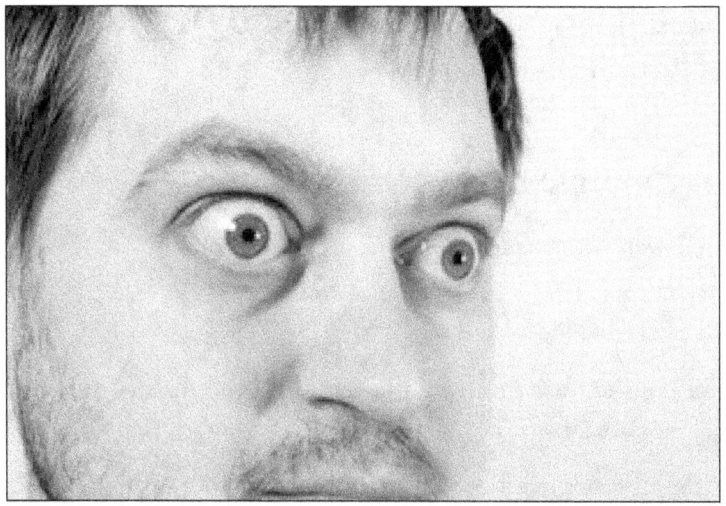

This is another topic that deserves a quick discussion.

Exophthalmos, or bulging of one or both eyes, occurs in about 30% of Graves' disease patients.

Graves' disease causes an enlargement in the extraocular muscles, swelling, and expansion of the orbital fat cells. Since there is limited space in the bony orbit, the only place for the eye to move is out.

About two-thirds of cases will resolve within six months once the hyperthyroidism is treated.[38]

Unfortunately, for the other one-third, the gradual protrusion of the eyeballs can continue even after treatment of their hyperthyroidism. In those cases, corticosteroids, chemotherapy agents, or even surgery may be needed.

I recommend that all patients who notice any bulging of their eyes be evaluated by an ophthalmologist for treatment and to rule out other potential causes besides thyroid eye disease.

CAN GRAVES' DISEASE BE CURED?

The answer to that question is another question. How do you define cure?

If you consider a cure to be the removal of all excess thyroid hormone, then RAI therapy and thyroidectomy definitely would meet that definition since both treatments remove any functioning thyroid gland.

Unfortunately, these treatments also mean a lifelong need for thyroid hormone medication.

If you define cure as optimal TSH, free T4, and free T3 levels in the absence of any thyroid medication or other medications, then very few Graves' patients will ever be cured.

Stopping antithyroid drugs such as methimazole is followed by a 50% recurrence of hyperthyroidism within four years.

In one study, at a 20-year follow-up of Graves' patients who had been treated with antithyroid drugs, only about 27% had a complete, permanent remission.[37]

In other words, unless you had RAI therapy or a thyroidectomy, there is a high likelihood that you will have a recurrence of Graves' disease at some point in your life.

Regular thyroid lab work, including TSI levels, TSH, free T4, and free T3, will be critical to monitor your thyroid function.

SUMMARY

- The causes of hyperthyroidism include Graves' disease, toxic nodules, thyroiditis, pituitary adenomas, thyroid cancer, and excessive thyroid medication.
- Graves' disease is the most common cause of hyperthyroidism. It is an autoimmune disease.
- Graves' disease is typically caused by a genetic predisposition that is activated by some type of trigger. These triggers include infections, gut dysbiosis, environmental toxins, food sensitivities, excessive iodine uptake, and stress.
- Common symptoms of hyperthyroid and Graves' disease include tremors, palpitations, hair loss, weight loss, diarrhea, fatigue, insomnia, and bulging eyes.

- Graves' disease is diagnosed via thyroid lab tests and thyroid antibody testing, thyroid ultrasound, and radioactive iodine uptake and scan testing.
- Conventional treatment for Graves' disease included anti-thyroid medication, radioactive iodine ablation, and removal of the thyroid (thyroidectomy).
- Natural treatments can help reduce symptoms and even lead to spontaneous remission in some people. These treatments include diet, targeted supplements, improvement of gut function, and stress reduction.
- Other treatments can include low-dose naltrexone and add-back therapy.
- Thyroid eye disease can occur in 30% of Graves' disease patients. If bulging of the eyes occurs, the patient should be evaluated by an ophthalmologist for treatment and to rule out other causes.
- 27% of Graves' disease patients may have spontaneous remission.

7.

THYROIDECTOMY AND RADIOACTIVE IODINE ABLATION

"Samuel" is a 43-year-old active male who asked to speak to me about his thyroid situation.

His journey began about two years earlier when he found himself tired and feeling foggy, with little energy, and overall worn out. He took an international trip to Africa in November, thinking that the solution to his fatigue was a little time away. Coming back from the trip, his symptoms persisted, so he sought medical counsel. At first, his doctor understandably assumed his symptoms were from his trip, so he was tested for everything from West Nile Virus to malaria. On the second visit, he was prescribed a broad-spectrum antibiotic and was told that maybe he had a sinus infection. On the third visit, he was given an anti-inflammatory and had further blood work. His TSH was 0. Three months later, he was finally diagnosed with hyperthyroidism. He was referred to an endocrinologist who started him on Methimazole.

It was another nine weeks before he was diagnosed with Graves' Disease. During that time, he had symptoms that included a 30-pound weight loss, heart palpitations, severe sweating, tremors, insomnia, fatigue, and others. The next few months were brutal. His endocrinologist would increase his methimazole and beta-blocker slowly, but it didn't seem to help. Further workup ensued, which also showed adrenal insufficiency. He was given more meds, which helped his symptoms only slightly. Within a few months, he felt progressively tired and short of breath. He was sent to a cardiologist who diagnosed him with high-output heart failure. After discussing everything with his endocrinologist, he made the decision to have a thyroidectomy almost a year after his first symptoms developed.

He was prescribed Synthroid for the next ten months. He never felt as good as he expected, so he was changed to a natural desiccated thyroid. His symptoms substantially improved on that medication.

People without a thyroid are just different than when they had a thyroid gland. If you have had yours removed or have had radioactive iodine ablation (RAIA), you probably feel a lot different than you did before your treatment.

They have typically gained a lot of weight, feel cold, constipated, fatigued, and have hair loss. Even if they are on thyroid medication, they still probably don't feel as good as they would like. Why? Let's break it down.

If you have had a thyroidectomy or RAIA treatment, there are some things to keep in mind:

1. You now have hypothyroidism - Chances are, if you have had your thyroid removed or destroyed by radioactive iodine (RAIA), it was because you were **hyper**thyroid. Now that your thyroid is gone (or destroyed), you have no thyroid function, and you are officially **hypo**thyroid.

It may take a few months for all the excess thyroid hormone to be depleted in your body, but it will eventually happen, and you will develop severe hypothyroid symptoms without aggressive treatment with thyroid medication.

It could even be deadly without treatment.

By the way, this also holds true for someone who has end-stage Hashimoto's thyroiditis. The thyroid gland becomes so atrophic and damaged that it no longer produces thyroid hormone.

Even if early in the disease process, Hashimoto's caused you to have periods of hyperthyroidism, that will no longer be the case once it is destroyed by the autoimmune antibodies.

It is effectively the same as if the thyroid gland had been removed.

2. You will be on thyroid medication for life - At this point in modern medicine, we don't have the ability to re-grow the thyroid gland. Once it is removed or completely destroyed, the only way to get thyroid hormone in your body is to take thyroid medication. That will be the case for the rest of your life.

In other chapters, I discussed how some people can potentially get off medication if they make changes to their diet, supplements, and lifestyle. That is NOT the case for people who have had a thyroidectomy or have no functional thyroid. Medication will always be needed.

3. T4-only medication is likely not enough for you - When a thyroid gland is surgically removed, completely killed from RAIA treatment, or is completely destroyed by long-standing Hashimoto's, it no longer produces thyroid hormone.

Most hypothyroid patients still have some thyroid gland production; they just can't produce enough on their own to reach optimal levels. Thyroid medication is needed to make up the difference from what the body is not producing itself.

As a reminder, a functioning thyroid gland produces mostly T4, but it also produces some T3 (and even T2).

Without any T3 production from the thyroid gland, all T3 hormone must come from the conversion of T4.

One study showed that everyone is different in how well they convert T4 to T3 in the peripheral tissues (that's what I have been screaming from the rooftops!).[1] When patients were given a T4-only medication, more than 20% were not able to achieve optimal levels of free T3 and free T4.

As you would expect, their free T4 levels were high, but their free T3 levels were low. They didn't feel as good as they should or could.

People without a functioning thyroid gland are deficient in BOTH T4 and T3. If over 20% of them don't convert T4 to T3 adequately, can you see why giving a T4-only medication such as levothyroxine wouldn't be enough?

Most people will feel better and have better thyroid hormone levels if they take <u>both</u> T4 and T3. This can be either as a natural desiccated thyroid medication or by adding liothyronine to their levothyroxine.

4. Weight gain is likely, and it will be even harder to lose weight - Studies show that about 80% of people who have their thyroid removed will gain weight. This can mean a weight gain of 15-20 pounds or even more.[2]

Why does this happen?

The primary reason is because their hypothyroidism is inadequately treated. They are typically put on levothyroxine or Synthroid, plus the dose is usually not high enough.

Even in the best of situations, weight loss is difficult after having your thyroid removed. It's not impossible, however. Proper medication and dosage, supplements, diet, and exercise can all be used to keep you at a healthy weight. See Chapter 10 and 11 for more information.

5. Thyroid supplements are still important - This can be a point of confusion for some people. If they no longer have a thyroid, then they think they don't need thyroid supplements.

This is completely false!

Remember, your doctor most likely put you on only one medication (levothyroxine), and that medication is not active.

So, what activates it? Deiodinase enzymes that are dependent on certain nutrients such as iodine, selenium, and many others. See Chapter 1 for more information.

Even though you no longer make thyroid hormone, you may still be deficient in some nutrients that are needed for normal cellular function.

For example, your body needs selenium for proper immune, antioxidant, and thyroid function. The skin and breast tissue still need iodine.

What are the most important nutrients for someone without a thyroid gland?

- Iodine
- Selenium
- Zinc
- Vitamin D
- Iron
- Adrenal Support
- Vitamin B12
- Magnesium
- Probiotics

A deficiency of one or more of these will prevent the body from operating at an optimalmlevel.

SUMMARY

- Thyroidectomy, RAIA, and long-standing Hashimoto's thyroiditis result in thyroid removal or complete destruction of the thyroid gland. They all result in permanent hypothyroidism.

- A large percentage of people have issues with T4 to T3 conver-sion. Replacing their thyroid hormone with T4-only medica-tion will likely be inadequate to resolve all of their hypothyroid symptoms.

- Weight gain is common after thyroidectomy or RAIA treatments. Weight loss is difficult but not impossible. Taking the right type and dose of thyroid medication is crucial to help you lose weight and keep it off.

- Thyroid supplements are important for all thyroidectomy and RAIA patients. Iodine, selenium, zinc, vitamin D, adrenal supple-ments, and others are essential to keep the cells of your body functioning properly and to ensure optimal deiodinase activity.

8.

THYROID NODULES AND OTHER DIFFICULT THYROID CASES

"Laura" is a 65-year-old female who presented to the office complaining of feeling terrible.

She was having severe fatigue, constipation, cold intolerance, swelling of her legs and face, hair loss, and a 30-pound weight gain over the past few years.

She already had a diagnosis of hypothyroidism and was taking levothy-roxine 0.1 mg daily. Her initial last tests showed a high TSH and low free T4 and free T3.

Her levothyroxine dose was gradually increased every 1-2 months until her symptoms began to improve. She started losing weight, and her energy increased dramatically.

At that time, her TSH was mildly suppressed, but her free T4 and free T3 levels were still slightly lower than optimal.

Her levothyroxine dose was 350 mcg daily!

A few months later, she went to the ER after having a minor car accident. The ER doctor saw her high levothyroxine dose and was shocked. He instructed her to stop all levothyroxine immediately because that much thyroid medication was "dangerous."

When she returned to my office a month later, she was having swelling in her face and legs, severe fatigue, and had gained almost 20 pounds.

Her TSH was almost 300! Free T4 was below measurable levels, and free T3 was 0.8.

She was immediately restarted on thyroid medication, and the dose was aggressively titrated until she was back on her previous dose.

THYROID NODULES

Thyroid nodules are extremely common, occurring in 4 to 7% of the population.[1]

Simply put, a thyroid nodule is a piece of tissue in your thyroid gland that is different from the surrounding tissue.[2]

Instead of the spongy, uniform texture of the thyroid gland, nodules typically have a different texture than the sounding thyroid tissue. Some may even be tender to the touch.

Most are discovered because they become visible externally, or they are found by either the medical provider or the patient when they palpate their anterior neck.

Others are found serendipitously from an imaging study, such as a chest CT or a neck ultrasound. These nodules vary in both size and consistency.

Older female patients get thyroid nodules more commonly than other populations. Statistically, more than 94% of all thyroid nodules are benign.[3]

Even though the chance of malignancy is low, all thyroid nodules should still be fully evaluated when they are discovered, which I will discuss in detail later in the chapter.

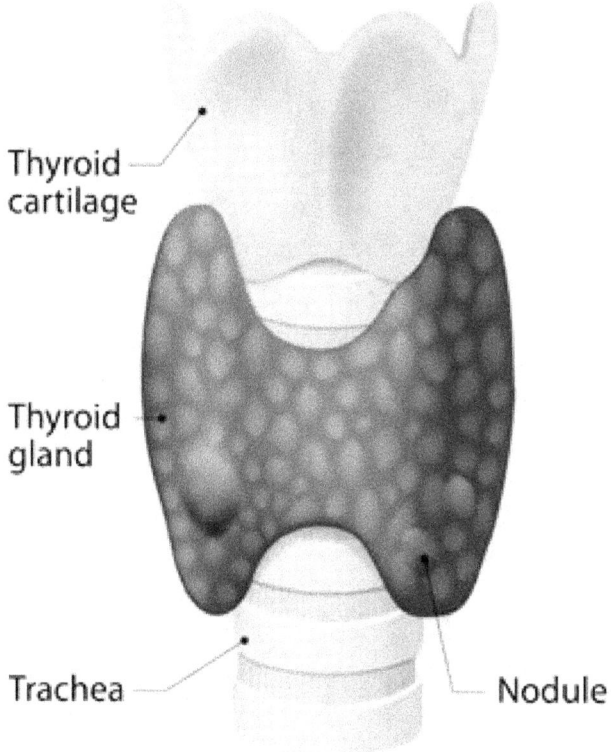

Thyroid cartilage

Thyroid gland

Trachea

Nodule

WHAT CAUSES THYROID NODULES?

In some cases, the cause can be identified, but in many cases, it's not clear. Known causes of thyroid nodules include:

- **Overgrowth of thyroid gland tissue** - This is probably the most common cause of thyroid nodules.

We aren't sure what causes the overgrowth, but it may have something to do with a combination of genetics, diet, nutrient deficiency, and environmental triggers.

- **Iodine deficiency** - Prior to the early 1900s, this was the most common cause worldwide.

With the iodization of salt and even water supplies, iodine deficiency is much less common but can still occur.

Iodine is primarily found in sea vegetables and iodized salt, so if your diet is lacking in either, there is a good chance you could be deficient.

Pregnant and nursing women also have a higher demand for iodine than other adults.

- **Thyroiditis** - Any condition that results in chronic inflammation can result in tissue overgrowth, scarring, and cancer.[4]

That is certainly the case in the thyroid of patients with Hashimoto's or Graves' disease.

Both of these autoimmune conditions are common and may be one of the reasons for the high incidence of thyroid nodules.

- **Thyroid cancer** - Although I have discussed the possibility of thyroid cancer developing over a long period of time due to one of the other conditions listed, sometimes cancer develops suddenly in the thyroid and can lead to nodules very quickly.

That is why all thyroid nodules need to be evaluated as soon as they are found.

- **Radiation exposure** - Radiation exposure is known to cause cellular damage and may precipitate thyroid nodule formation.

Radiation dose and exposure increase the risk for both thyroid nodules and cancer.[5]

The thyroid gland is extremely sensitive to radiation. That is why patients who have been exposed to radiation are treated with high doses of iodine.

WHAT SYMPTOMS DO THYROID NODULES CAUSE?

Most thyroid nodules are asymptomatic and are only discovered because they are either visible on an external exam, are found by palpating the anterior neck, or are found accidentally from a test such as a chest CT scan or a neck ultrasound.

Occasionally, however, patients may experience changes in their thyroid function, which will result in symptoms.

If the nodule produces excessive thyroid hormone, the typical symptoms of <u>hyperthyroidism</u> may be present—palpitations, tremors, sweating, insomnia, anxiety, weight loss, and diarrhea.

If the nodule suppresses normal thyroid function in the surrounding thyroid tissue, symptoms of <u>hypothyroidism</u> will result—fatigue, hair loss, weight gain, constipation, dry skin, brain fog, and depression.

If the nodule is large or cancerous, it can compress other neck structures or result in lymph node enlargement that can lead to these symptoms—pain when swallowing, hoarseness, difficulty breathing, or pain in the thyroid gland.

MEDICAL WORKUP FOR THYROID NODULES

If a thyroid nodule is discovered, the next step is to undergo testing.

Testing takes the form of lab testing and a thyroid ultrasound.

Thyroid labs are checked to see how well the thyroid gland is working. Is there any hypothyroidism or hyperthyroidism?

A thyroid ultrasound is also performed to directly image the thyroid gland and give key information about the size and other characteristics of the nodule and thyroid tissue.[6]

There are certain findings that may increase the likelihood of thyroid cancer:

- Nodules larger than 4 cm
- Firmness of the nodule (the more firm, the higher the risk)
- Fixation of the nodule to surrounding tissue
- Enlarged lymph nodes in the neck or near the nodule
- Hoarseness or changes to the vocal cords
- Microcalcifications on ultrasound
- The absence of a "halo" on ultrasound
- Hypoechoic on ultrasound
- Increased nodule flow on ultrasound

If one or more of these findings are present, a fine needle aspiration (FNA) should be ordered to biopsy the nodule.

Unfortunately, up to 25% of FNA biopsies may give an "inconclusive" result. In these cases, the nodule is monitored at regular intervals and may be biopsied again at a future date if an ultrasound or exam shows any changes in size or texture.

A radioactive iodine uptake (RIAU) scan may also be ordered.

In this test, a predetermined amount of radioactive iodine will be consumed.

Since iodine is absorbed by the thyroid gland, scans can be ordered at periodic intervals to determine the amount of radioactive iodine that was absorbed by the thyroid gland and the nodule in particular.

If the nodule is "hot" (takes up a large amount of the radioactive iodine), then it is producing excessive amounts of thyroid hormone. This is typical of nodules caused by Hashimoto's and Graves' disease.

If the nodule is "cold" (doesn't absorb any radioactive iodine), then it is not producing thyroid hormone and could actually suppress the surrounding thyroid tissue and keep it from producing normal thyroid hormone amounts. Cold nodules are especially concerning for malignancy and are usually biopsied.

TREATMENT OF THYROID NODULES

There are three basic ways of treating a thyroid nodule: You can remove it, monitor it, or try to shrink it.

1. Removal - In most cases, it is not necessary to remove the thyroid nodule unless it is cancerous or produces excessive thyroid hormone.

2. Monitor - The majority of thyroid nodules are treated this way.

This includes regular visits to your medical provider for physical exams and lab testing.

It will also require getting thyroid ultrasounds at regular intervals to monitor for any changes in the nodule over time.

If there are changes noticed, either removal or biopsy will likely be recommended.

3. Attempt to shrink the nodule - Many patients are interested in this treatment option.

Whether this option will work depends in large part on the cause of the nodule.

If the nodule is due to iodine deficiency, it can be easily treated by taking an iodine supplement.

If the nodule is due to thyroid tissue overgrowth, shrinking may be possible but more difficult.

Studies have shown that high levels of TSH may be stimulating to the thyroid gland tissue and may increase the growth of thyroid nodules and thyroid cancer.[7]

For this reason, some providers will treat thyroid cancer by giving suppressive doses of thyroid hormone medication.[8]

Taking thyroid medication will block TSH production from the pituitary gland.

Although this concept is not commonly used to treat non-cancerous thyroid nodules, some of the information can be used to devise natural therapies that could help.

If we can increase normal thyroid production, we could naturally reduce TSH levels.

Natural therapies that may help treat thyroid nodules include:

- Supplementing with zinc and selenium
- Optimizing T4 to T3 conversion through supplements, diet, exercise, and other lifestyle changes.
- Taking thyroid medication (T4/T3)
- Reducing inflammation in the body
- Optimizing immune function
- Reducing stress (yoga, meditation, etc.)

Obviously, natural treatments aren't guaranteed to work, but at the very least, they have the potential to get your body in a more healthy state, which will only help the situation.

SOME DIFFICULT CASES

Sometimes, the symptoms and lab results for someone just don't make sense.

There are some rare genetic defects that can affect thyroid receptor function and sensitivity to thyroid hormones.

If you are a patient with one of these issues, getting proper treatment is going to be extremely difficult, so you need to understand what is going on in your body.

If you are a medical provider and have one of these patients come to see you, then it may be extremely confusing how to manage them.

- Pituitary Adenomas

Let's look at another patient story.

A 40-year-old female came to the clinic asking for help.

She was having severe hypothyroid symptoms, including weight gain, constipation, hair loss, depression, and crippling fatigue. She also had very irregular menstrual cycles.

Here are her lab results:

TSH				
TSH	0.008	Low	uIU/mL	0.450-4.500
T4,Free(Direct)	<0.10	Low	ng/dL	0.82-1.77
Triiodothyronine (T3), Free				
Triiodothyronine (T3), Free	0.7	Low	pg/mL	2.0-4.4

These results don't make sense, do they?

If TSH is low, free hormone levels should be high and vice-versa, right? Something else must be going on.

In this particular case, she had a pituitary adenoma that was suppressing her normal TSH production. With a low TSH level, her thyroid was not getting the signal to produce thyroid hormone.

Other clues to a pituitary adenoma can be abnormalities in other hormone systems, such as the adrenal and sex hormones. If there is a growth that is suppressing TSH production, it is likely also suppressing ACTH and FSH levels.

When those hormone levels are suppressed in the pituitary, that usually results in an elevated prolactin level.

Any time there are abnormally low levels of any of the stimulating hormones, a prolactin level should be tested.

- Thyroid Resistance

There is also a syndrome called Thyroid Resistance Syndrome.

Thyroid resistance is caused by the body's tissues being resistant to the effects of thyroid hormone.

Thyroid resistance is predominantly an inherited condition that occurs in one out of every 40,000 births.[9]

It is usually caused by a genetic mutation that results in the thyroid hormone receptors being defective.

It affects both men and women equally and can occur at any age.

The abnormal thyroid receptors do not respond to thyroid hormones, especially in the pituitary gland, so typically, the TSH levels remain high in spite of high circulating free thyroid hormone levels.

They can present with either hypothyroid or hyperthyroid symptoms.

In these cases, treating their symptoms and clinical picture should be the focus, not the thyroid lab results.

TSH-producing pituitary tumors can present with similar thyroid lab results, so a workup should be done on anyone who presents with confusing results.

The clinical case presented at the start of this chapter is yet another example of someone with thyroid resistance.

In her case, her pituitary responded appropriately to thyroid hormones, but the peripheral cells of her body didn't.

Supraphysiologic doses of thyroid hormone medications were required to keep her T4 and T3 levels near normal ranges.

SUMMARY

- Thyroid nodules are fairly common, occurring in up to 7% of the US population.

- Most are asymptomatic and are only discovered because they can be seen externally or palpated in the neck or are found on an im-aging test that was ordered for another reason.

- Several things are known to cause thyroid nodules. These include overgrowth of thyroid tissue, iodine deficiency, thyroiditis, thy-roid cancer, and radiation exposure.

- Any patient with a thyroid nodule should have thyroid lab test-ing and a thyroid ultrasound performed. Depending on those results, radioactive iodine uptake scans and even fine needle aspi-ration may be needed.

- Treatment of thyroid nodules can involve surgical removal, moni-toring over time, or even attempting to shrink the nodule through the use of suppressive thyroid medication and natural therapies such as diet, lifestyle changes, and targeted supplements.

- If thyroid lab results don't make sense, look for less common con-ditions such as pituitary adenomas or thyroid resistance.

- In thyroid resistance, it is more important to treat the symptoms of the patient rather than treating based on the lab results.

9.

THYROID MEDICATION: CURRENTLY AVAILABLE OPTIONS AND HOW TO OPTIMIZE THEIR USE

"Cindy" is a 58-year-old female who asked me to start managing her hypothyroidism.

She had been diagnosed around ten years earlier. At that time, she told her gynecologist that she had been feeling more tired than usual, and her hair seemed to be thinning. After checking some screening lab work, her TSH was found to be elevated (I don't know at what level).

She was prescribed levothyroxine 0.05 mg daily.

She had little to no improvement in her symptoms, but her doctor would not change or increase the medication because he said her TSH was now "normal."

After checking a complete thyroid panel, I found her TSH to be slightly elevated at 2.63, free T4 was 0.9, her free T3 level was low at 2.5, her reverse T3 level slightly high at 14.2, and her TPO antibody level was high at 63.

I stopped her levothyroxine and started her on Armour Thyroid 30 mg daily. After four weeks, I increased her dose to 60 mg daily. I also started her on selenium, adrenal adaptogens, and a multivitamin. I encouraged her to remove gluten and dairy from her diet. We also discussed proper sleep hygiene, stress management, and the importance of regular exercise.

Two months later, we rechecked her lab work, which showed a TSH of 0.95, free T4 of 0.97, a free T3 level of 3.5, a reverse T3 of 9.3, and a TPO antibody level of 52.

She felt much better than she had in many years and was having no side effects from her new medication and supplements.

There is a good chance that when someone thinks of thyroid medication, the only one that comes to mind is Synthroid or levothyroxine. However, there are many other brands and types to choose from.

In this chapter, I will discuss the various thyroid medications that are available, as well as tips on when it is best to use which ones.

Thyroid medications primarily differ in three major areas:
- How much thyroid hormone they contain
- Which thyroid hormones they contain
- What fillers and binders they contain

All these areas can impact how well you tolerate the medication and how well it works in your body.

Knowing this information could be invaluable in helping you find the right medication to treat your thyroid condition with the least possible side effects.

As a reminder, there are two main types of thyroid hormone found in your body—T4 and T3. T2 and even T1 are also present but at much lower levels than the other two.

T4 is the most common thyroid hormone in your body. Think of it as the "transport" form of thyroid. It is very stable but has very little thyroid function itself. It must be converted to T3 to become active.

T3 is the most active form of thyroid. Its free form is what directly binds to the cells of the body to trigger the metabolic functions within the cells.

When the system is functioning normally, the thyroid gland will produce a steady stream of thyroid hormone at a ratio of about 80% T4 to 20% T3.[1]

Since that ratio is normally found in the human body, it is usually the ratio you should try to achieve when using thyroid medication. However, there are many instances where it may need to be different to achieve the best results for a particular person.

There are many different thyroid medications available in the US (and even more in other countries). Let's break them down further.

T4-ONLY THYROID MEDICATION

- Synthroid
- Levothyroxine
- Tirosint
- Levoxyl
- Levothroid
- Unithroid
- Euthyrox
- Levo-T

These are the most commonly prescribed of all thyroid medications. In fact, Synthroid is one of the most commonly prescribed medications in the United States.

They are considered extremely stable and the "safest" thyroid medications to take. If you miss a dose, take too much, or make any other mistake with the medications, the consequences are generally not dangerous.

Unfortunately, they simply may not be adequate to properly treat a lot of thyroid patients.

Studies have shown that up to 20% of people taking T4-only medication may still experience hypothyroid symptoms despite taking "sufficient" amounts of thyroid medication.[2]

This group of people typically have an issue with converting T4 to T3. This can either be due to genetic variations or conditions that impair the conversion.

These include nutrient deficiencies (iodine, selenium, zinc, vitamin D) and chronic inflammatory conditions (insulin resistance, autoimmunity, chronic illness, etc.).

If you feel worse after taking levothyroxine or Synthroid, it could be that you are reacting to a filler or other component that is in the pill.

These fillers do not contain active medication but do things such as stabilize the medication, regulate medication release, change the color of the pill, etc.

Even though they are thought to be "inert," studies have shown that they can cause issues for many patients.[3] This is especially true for thyroid patients, who tend to be more sensitive to substances than patients without thyroid issues.

Symptoms that can be caused by fillers in medication include bloating, diarrhea, constipation, runny nose, headache, swelling, rash, and itching.

Many of these symptoms are non-specific and can be caused by a multitude of things.

That is why it is very important to pay attention to when your symptoms started and if they correlate with when you started your thyroid medication.

An example of one of these fillers is lactose monohydrate. It can block the absorption of levothyroxine and can even cause resistance to levothyroxine in patients with lactose intolerance.[4]

This is especially important in patients with Hashimoto's. Removing lactose from their diet has been shown to improve thyroid function.[5] I don't know why it is still used as a filler in some products.

Gluten can potentially be found in small amounts in some generic levothyroxine medication, so be sure to talk to your pharmacist about that if you have a history of gluten sensitivity or allergy.

Tirosint is a T4-only medication that can be very beneficial for patients with multiple allergies or sensitivities to food or medications.

If you suspect you could be reacting to a filler in your thyroid medication, it might be worth trying Tirosint.

Tirosint only contains thyroxine, gelatin, water, and glycerin, making it the cleanest thyroid medication on the market.

It also absorbs better than other thyroid medications. Studies have shown that it can be absorbed even when taking it with food and/or coffee.[6] For someone who struggles taking their thyroid medication on an empty stomach, Tirosint may be a good choice.

Keep in mind that Tirosint is substantially more expensive than generic levothyroxine. It may even be difficult to get medical insurance to cover it. Some companies have started producing generic versions of Tirosint, so hopefully, the price will continue to decrease.

Normal therapeutic doses for T4-only medications are anywhere from 50 mcg daily to around 200 mcg daily. Patients with thyroid resistance may even need substantially higher doses.

NATURAL DESICCATED THYROID (NDT) MEDICATION

- Armour Thyroid
- NP Thyroid
- WP Thyroid
- Nature-Throid
- Thyrolar
- Adthyza

There are other names for NDT medications in other countries, but these medications share one thing in common: They are produced from desiccated glands of animals.

What does that mean?

These medications are created by drying and crushing the thyroid glands of animals (usually pigs) and then formulating them into medication.

They are unique among all thyroid medications because they contain much more than just thyroid hormones. Since it contains the entire thyroid gland of animals, they also contain trace amounts of other nutrients, less active forms of thyroid hormone, proteins, and minerals.

The way they are dosed is also different from other thyroid medications. They are split up into what is referred to as "grains."

Each grain of NDT contains a standardized amount of T4 and T3. This helps to ensure that you always get the same amount of thyroid hormone regardless of which brand you are using.

Each grain of NDT contains 38 micrograms of T4 hormone and 9 mcg of T3 hormone.[7]

Remember to count the grains and not the milligrams when changing from one brand of NDT to another.

For example, 60 mg of Armour Thyroid and Nature-Throid 65 mg both contain one grain of NDT, as does 65 mg of Adthyza.

NDT meds are a great starting point if you have not responded well to T4 medications in the past or if you have a low free T3 and high reverse T3 lab result.

A typical therapeutic dose for most patients is 30 mg to 150 mg daily.

On a side note, there are various NDT-like thyroid supplements available on the market. Eco Thyro and Spark Plug are examples. They contain concentrated thyroid tissue. They are available over the counter and typically come in only one or two different strengths.

Many supplement producers do not follow the stringent production regulations of the prescription pharmaceutical industry. There is a risk of the thyroid hormone content varying from bottle to bottle. Due to that and the limited dosages available, I do not recommend the use of these products.

Please let your medical provider know if you are taking one of them because it can drastically affect your thyroid medication and dosage.

T3-ONLY MEDICATIONS

- Cytomel
- Liothyronine
- Sustained-release (SR) T3

T3-only medications are the strongest type of thyroid hormone medication available.

These medications are not commonly prescribed by most conventional medicine providers because they assume that the body can convert T4 to T3 without any issues.

Hopefully, by now, I have convinced you that this is not the case for a lot of people.

Many thyroid patients may potentially benefit greatly from taking a T3-only medication, effectively bypassing the need for the body to convert it from T4.

Unfortunately, most medical providers have little to no experience using them, which makes them uncomfortable prescribing them. Many may also express concerns about possible side effects from T3-only medications, such as palpitations, atrial fibrillation, and bone loss.

In my experience, about 25-30% of people who start liothyronine or Cytomel experience mild side effects from taking it—mostly jitteriness or anxiety symptoms. In most cases, the symptoms will resolve after a few days. It can also help to cut the dose in half and take it twice or more throughout the day.

When used in appropriate amounts and when patients are monitored closely, there should be minimal to no risk for atrial fibrillation.

In fact, studies have shown that both hypothyroidism and hyperthyroidism increase the incidence of atrial fibrillation.[8]

If your hypothyroidism is not optimally treated on a T4-only medication, that is likely more of a risk for the development of atrial fibrillation than adding a T3 medication to your regimen.

So, what about bone density?

It is likely that some of you have been told something like this: "Your TSH is too low. We need to back off your thyroid medication, or you could develop osteoporosis."

While there are some studies that show longstanding Graves' disease can result in loss of bone mass, this study showed that suppressing the TSH with high levels of thyroid medication for up to three years did not have any impact on their bone density.[9]

Free hormone levels should be used to determine thyroid hormone levels, not TSH.

If someone is taking thyroid medication and their free T3 level is in the optimal range, then they are NOT hyperthyroid, even if their TSH is suppressed.

If their free T3 levels are above the optimal range, I would recommend reducing their dose. Getting people to their optimal thyroid levels should be the goal for everyone.

Cytomel comes in unusual strengths—5 mcg, 25 mcg, and 50 mcg.

Typically, I start patients on 5 or 10 mcg, then titrate up slowly every few weeks as necessary. Most patients ultimately need a dose in the 25 mcg to 50 mcg range.

If side effects from the short-acting T3 medications persist, it may be necessary to switch to a sustained-release T3. This medication must be produced from a compounding pharmacy and will not be available in a conventional retail pharmacy.

COMPOUNDED T4 AND T3 THYROID MEDICATION

These medications are not available in a standard pharmacy. They can only be made in a compounding pharmacy.

A compounding pharmacy can create a medication onsite that is unique to any particular need.[10]

They can make a medication using different inactive ingredients that can be applied to the skin instead of taken orally, etc.

This is especially valuable when making thyroid medication.

If your body needs a different T4 to T3 ratio than the typical 80/20, a compounding pharmacy can make it to the specifications needed for a particular patient.

Also, compounding pharmacies can make T3 medication in a sustained-release form. This allows for the medication to be released gradually over time instead of having a large amount of the hormone enter the bloodstream all at once. This can help reduce the side effects that many people have with Cytomel (liothyronine).

Unfortunately, compounding pharmacies are typically more expensive than traditional pharmacies. For instance, your compounded thyroid medication may cost around $50 per month instead of the typical $4-$10 per month of the standard thyroid medications.

They are also not covered by health insurance plans.

Many medical providers are unfamiliar with using compounding pharmacies or selecting the correct thyroid doses. It will be important for you to find someone with experience in thyroid management if you want to consider compounded thyroid medication. I will discuss how to do this in Chapter 12.

HOW TO OPTIMIZE YOUR THYROID MEDICATION

If you are taking your thyroid medication faithfully every day but still experiencing low thyroid symptoms, there are some things you can do to get an optimal response.

Some of these will require a medical provider who is willing to work with you. Some you will be able to do on your own.

1. Change the thyroid medication you are taking

Most people do better and feel better when they use a combination of T4 and T3.

As I have stated, conventional medicine only recommends using T4-only thyroid medication. In other words, 100% T4.

Essentially, every thyroid patient will have a different ratio of T4/T3 where they feel the best.

One might feel great on 100% T4, while another does better with 80% T4 and 20% T3, and yet another does best on 50% T4 and 50% T3.

The only way to find out where you or your patient feels best is to change the ratio.

For someone who isn't feeling great on their medication, they would likely benefit from trying some of the different thyroid formulations—Tirosint, NDT, liothyronine in addition to their T4-only medication, or even compounded T4/T3 medication.

Thyroid management is not an exact science. Adjusting dosages and/or types of medication will likely be necessary to find the optimal treatment program for each person.

2. Change how you take your thyroid medication

The vast majority of thyroid patients take their medication orally with water. They are instructed to avoid taking other medications/supplements/food both before and after their thyroid medicine.

While this works great for most people, some might benefit from other options.

Mashing up your thyroid tablet and placing it under your tongue (sublingual) can be beneficial for some patients with absorption issues.

If your medication is in gel cap form, then opening the capsule and squeezing it directly under the tongue is also an option.

In rare instances, when patients have severe GI absorption issues, it is even possible to do thyroid medicine injections, although I personally have no experience with this.

3. Consider taking your thyroid medication at a different time
Although almost all medical providers and pharmacists recommend that patients take their thyroid medication first thing in the morning, right when they wake up and are away from food, it really isn't necessary to do that.

Taking it in the evening has actually been shown to be the best time of day.[11]

This may be better because intestinal function is usually slower in the evening, which will allow for better absorption.

Another option is to split your thyroid dosage into two or more different times throughout the day. This more closely mimics what a healthy thyroid gland would do.

This technique is particularly helpful for patients who are sensitive to T3 medication. Dividing into two or more doses will minimize the T3 load they receive each time and may minimize side effects from the T3.

For patients who are even sensitive to small dosing changes of levothyroxine, alternating daily total doses can help. For example, if someone is trying to increase their levothyroxine dose from 50 mcg to 75 mcg, it may help them to alternate taking the two strengths for a few weeks to help with the transition.

Even taking higher doses on the weekends or every third day are possibilities.

Really, it's simply a matter of trying different things until you figure out what works best for you.

4, Change your dose of thyroid medication

As I have stated previously, most medical providers only look at the TSH to determine a patient's thyroid dosage. If it is in the "normal" range, they assume that the thyroid dosage must be correct.

That is likely inadequate for many patients.

If you are still having symptoms of low thyroid, there is a high likelihood that you are on too low of a dose.

Your dosing needs can also change depending on what is going on in your life.

Factors such as age, other medical conditions, recent illness or infection, stress, other hormone levels, and how much you are sleeping can all affect how much thyroid hormone you need.

For this reason, you need to always pay attention to your symptoms and your thyroid lab tests to know if you need to adjust your medication dose.

Keep in mind that you can't determine if a dose is working for you or not unless you give it enough time.

Thyroid medication takes about six weeks to take effect in the body.

Changing it before that amount of time will only lead to inconsistent or even confusing results.

I don't recommend self-managing your thyroid dose without consulting and involving your medical provider.

If I have a knowledgeable patient who is very attuned to how they feel and will stay in communication with me, I will sometimes give them permission to do a gradual titration of their thyroid medication without having to contact me with each slight change.

In those situations, it is important to regularly check thyroid labs to make sure the patient isn't pushing the dose excessively.

Summary

- There are multiple thyroid medications currently available. They are primarily differentiated by their thyroid content but also by their fillers and binders.

- If someone isn't responding to a thyroid medication or is having side effects, it may be due to the fillers rather than the thyroid hormone itself.

- T4-only medications are the most commonly used and are generally very safe. However, if you have a T4 to T3 conversion issue, they may be inadequate to get you feeling optimal.

- If you think you are reacting to fillers in your T4 medication, it may be worth switching to Tirosint, which is much cleaner.

- NDT medications are a great option if T4 medications do not control your symptoms or if you have a high reverse T3 and low T3.

- T3-only medications are the most potent thyroid medicine available. They are generally well tolerated, but some people may be sensitive to them (mainly shaky, jittery, or a high heart rate). In that case, splitting the dose into two or more times per day can help, or using sustained-release compounded T3 may be needed.

- Other things that can be done to optimize your thyroid levels include taking your medication in the evening instead of the morning, splitting the dose, taking it two or more times per day, and even alternating strengths.

- Don't make thyroid medication changes more than every six weeks. It takes that long to equilibrate in your body. Changing more often will only confuse the results.

10.

WHY THYROID PATIENTS STRUGGLE LOSING WEIGHT

"Denise" is a 49-year-old female who consulted with me to help her lose weight. She had tried essentially every diet on the market over the years. She had even done ten cycles of the HCG diet. In the first cycle, she lost 20 pounds. Every cycle after that resulted in less weight loss. By the last few cycles, she couldn't lose any weight. She worked out at least five days per week but had reduced it to just walking because anything more than that completely exhausted her.

She even tried fasting for 22 hours every day for a month. She was eating a strict Paleo diet and never cheated. She was having to limit her calorie intake to only 500 calories per day just to maintain her current 175 pounds (she is 5'2" tall). If she even cheated a little bit, her weight would jump five or ten pounds within a few days. She was constantly stressed due to work and home issues. She was otherwise healthy and taking no medications.

Her lab work showed a "normal" TSH and free T4. Free T3 was low, reverse T3 extremely high, thyroid antibodies were negative, FSH was in the menopausal range, testosterone was suboptimal, and her morning cortisol was low. HgbA1c was great, but serum leptin was elevated at 77.

I diagnosed her with adrenal fatigue, menopause, hypothyroidism, leptin resistance, and metabolic damage from excessive calorie restriction.

She was treated with NDT thyroid, selenium 200 mcg daily, Zinc 30 mg daily, a methylated B vitamin, adrenal glandular and adaptogens, and a GLP-1 agonist. I explained that it would take months for her metabolism to recover. Despite her objections, I recommended that she eat a minimum of 1200 calories per day. I explained that she would likely gain ten or more pounds at first, but it was essential to "reset" her metabolism if she ever hoped to one day get her weight down into an ideal range. I also recommended testosterone and estrogen replacement therapy in the future once the other hormonal systems had improved. I explained that it could take six months or even a year to repair her metabolism enough that it would start responding to treatments.

Denise was very frustrated with my treatment recommendations, so she never followed back up with me. She could not bear the thought of potentially gaining ten or more pounds (ever if it was temporary).

I emailed her a few months later. At that time, she was still eating only 800 calories per day and was struggling to maintain her weight. I never saw her as a patient again.

One of the most frustrating aspects of thyroid disease is the weight gain and difficulty in losing weight that often comes with it. Why is that? What makes it so hard to lose weight when you have a thyroid condition?

There is neither an easy explanation nor an easy solution. But don't fret. It can be done if you are patient and committed to the process and if you work with a medical professional who has experience with such difficult cases.

Let's start by talking about weight loss in general. I will then explain how thyroid conditions can affect the whole process.

THE CALORIE IN, CALORIE OUT THEORY AND EAT LESS, EXERCISE MORE THEORY SIMPLY DON'T WORK

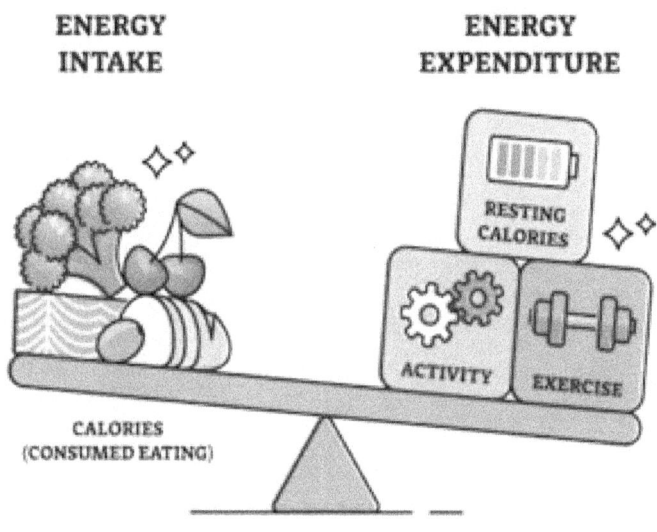

We have all (including doctors) been taught for years that weight loss should be simple and straightforward. As long as you consume fewer calories than you burn, you will lose weight.

In my training, I was taught to imagine a bucket that represents the body. There is a faucet at the bottom of the bucket and another faucet above the bucket. Water is coming out of both faucets.

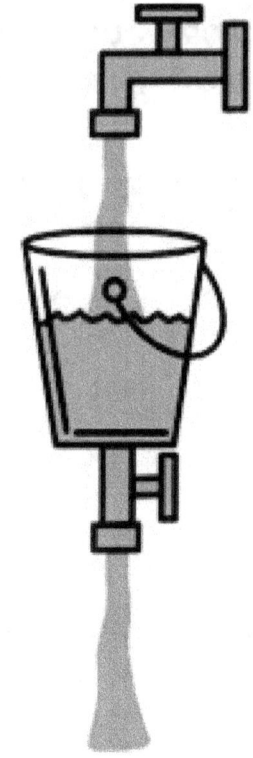

If the faucet that is pouring water into the bucket is pouring in more water than the faucet that is emptying water from the bucket, the bucket will slowly fill with water.

If the faucet that is pouring water into the bucket is pouring in less water than the faucet that is emptying water from the bucket, the bucket will slowly empty.

If the water flow from both faucets is equal, then the water level in the bucket will remain constant.

Now, imagine that the water represents calories.

That visual made perfect sense to me when it came to weight loss. People who are gaining weight are obviously consuming more calories than they are burning, which results in weight gain.

They just need to reduce their calories and exercise more, and the weight should come off easily.

Simple, right? There is just one problem...**It doesn't work.**

Most of you already intuitively know this. How many of you are eating very little and exercising as much as you can, but your weight doesn't budge?

A study from 1997 showed that between 1980 and 1990, Americans consumed about 4% fewer calories than in previous decades, yet the incidence of obesity increased by 31%[1]. They called it the "American Paradox."

A United Kingdom review from 2015 showed that the probability of achieving a normal weight by just reducing calories was 0.8% in women and 0.47% in men. In other words, losing weight by using the conventional calorie-counting methods had a failure rate of 99.2%![2]

Despite these findings, the medical establishment still embraces these incorrect concepts.

I was guilty of it earlier in my own career. When I saw a patient who was overweight and frustrated that they couldn't lose any weight, I typically responded with one of these statements:

- "You are probably eating more calories than you realize."
- "You need to increase the intensity of your exercise so you can burn off more calories."
- "I bet that you are cheating on your diet more than you think."

Yes, if you are consuming massive amounts of junk food daily, then you need to reduce your food intake. If you never get off the couch, then you need to start doing some exercise.

That doesn't describe a large percentage of people, however.

Many of the patients that I talk to have tried just about every fad diet on the market and have exercised above and beyond the recommended levels and intensity. Yet, their weight doesn't budge.

Counting calories and increasing exercise do not work for long-term weight loss.

In fact, reducing your calories too much for an extended period of time can actually be harmful to your metabolism.

THE PROBLEM WITH SEVERE CALORIE-RESTRICTED DIETS

Do you remember the TV show *The Biggest Loser?* It was a very popular show on NBC that ran from 2004 through 2016.

On the show, several contestants per season were put on severe calorie-restricted diets (about 800 calories per day) and intense exercise programs around eight hours per day for 30 weeks.

The show followed the contestants' journeys through the process.

Their weight loss was dramatic: Some of the contestants lost over 200 pounds by the end of the 30 weeks.

It really seemed to validate the "eat less, exercise more" philosophy.

Then, some researchers decided to follow up with some of the show's contestants.

Their findings were published in what is now called the Biggest Loser Study.

Fourteen contestants from the 2009 show were studied. All but one of them regained most, if not all, of the weight they had lost while on the show (plus sometimes even more) six years after the show.[3]

Instead of burning the typical ~2000 calories per day that they burned before being on the show, their resting metabolic rate dropped to about 1000 calories per day.

Even eating a meager 1200 calories per day would cause a gradual weight gain in the contestants.

In other words, the severe calorie-restricted diets that they were on during the show had severely damaged their metabolism.

The damage was still present six years later.

I have seen similar things in my medical practice.

Patients who have been on various severe calorie-restricted diets in the past (HCG diet and others) have presented to me with their metabolism in shambles.

Many of these poor people have to eat as little as 500 calories per day just to maintain their current weight (see the case study at the beginning of the chapter).

Their stories are similar: When they first went on severe calorie-restricted diets, they lost a ton of weight.

When they tried it again a few months later, they lost a little, but not as much as the first time.

When they tried it the last time, they lost little or no weight.

Their metabolism dropped each time they did the diet and didn't return to normal after they stopped.

They experienced what is described as **Metabolic Adaptation.**[4]

Their body responded to the continual low-calorie diet by going into starvation mode and reducing their metabolism. The body considered the low-calorie diet to be the "new normal."

Unfortunately, for those folks, the recovery process is going to be a long, frustrating road. It can be done, but it's not easy.

I will discuss weight loss strategies in the next chapter.

ROOT ISSUES CAUSING WEIGHT GAIN
AND PREVENTING WEIGHT LOSS

So, if "calories in, calories out" and "eat less, exercise more" are wrong, what are the real reasons that we can't lose weight?

As Dr. Jason Fung in *The Obesity Code* so succinctly states: The underlying cause of obesity is an imbalance of your hormones, NOT an imbalance of your calories![5]

The real root issue is hormone imbalance, particularly insulin resistance and leptin resistance, and/or thyroid disorders (or likely all the above).

In order to better understand this concept, it helps to look at the cascade of events that occur in the body when we eat (particularly sugar, carbs, and protein).

- After we eat, carbs and proteins are absorbed in the intestines, then the majority of them are transported immediately to the liver through the portal vein.
- This stimulates the pancreas to release insulin, which goes to the liver.
- Insulin binds to receptors on the cells of the liver, which opens channels that allow the sugar to enter the cells.
- The liver cells convert as much sugar as they can into glycogen, which it stores for future energy needs.
- Once the liver is full of glycogen, it then converts the remaining sugar and fructose into triglycerides (what is called lipogenesis).[6] Fructose must be converted to glucose and then to glycogen via gluconeogenesis, or it can be converted to triglycerides. It is easier just to convert it to triglycerides, so very little is converted to glycogen.
- The triglycerides are then released into the bloodstream, where they can be stored in adipocytes (fat cells) throughout the tissues of the body.
- To prevent overexpansion, when the fat cells become "full," they release leptin, which signals the hypothalamus that we need to stop eating and increase metabolism.
- The hypothalamus does this by stimulating the thyroid to release more thyroid hormone, which then signals the cells of the body to increase energy usage.
- The increase in leptin also triggers ghrelin levels to drop, which reduces appetite.[7]
- The increased energy expenditure burns off the excess fat in the fat cells, which then reduces their secretion of leptin.
- That is how the system works when everything is in balance.

If you are a layperson, this is probably more information than you want to know or understand. However, I believe it is important to at least have a cursory understanding of what is going on in the body.

So, what happens differently when someone is overweight or obese?

- The liver is constantly bombarded with more sugar than it can store as glycogen.
- The pancreas secretes even more insulin to try to drive the sugar out of the blood into the cells.
- The liver responds to the bombardment of insulin by reducing its response to it (insulin resistance).
- Lipogenesis increases to try to decrease the sugar and fructose in the blood.
- The fat cells then become bombarded by more and more triglycerides trying to be stored in them.
- The excess of fat in the fat cells signals them to release leptin at higher and higher amounts.
- The constant bombardment of the hypothalamus by high leptin levels causes it to decrease its response to the leptin (leptin resistance).
- The lack of response to leptin keeps the body locked in "starvation mode." Hunger levels remain high because when the hypothalamus ignores the leptin signal (due to leptin resistance), ghrelin levels stay elevated, and metabolism remains low (due to the impairment of normal thyroid function).
- The impaired thyroid function results in a decrease in metabolism, which leads to a direct negative effect on sugar and carbohydrate metabolism by worsening insulin resistance.[8, 9]
- The vicious cycle continues.

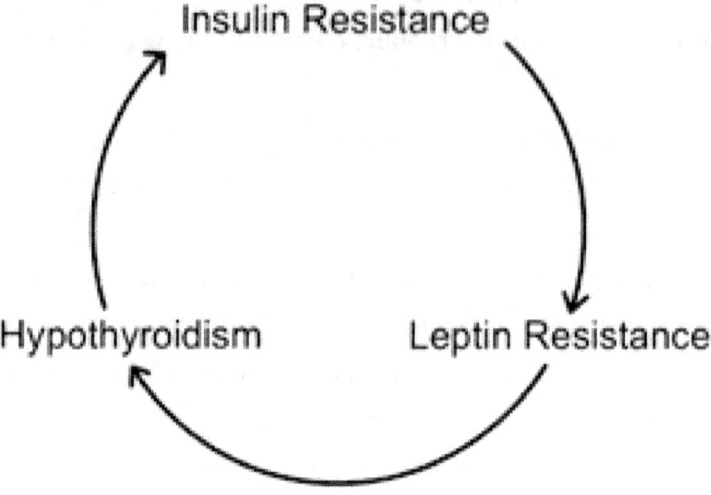

Fructose is even worse than glucose. It cannot be easily converted to glycogen, so the vast majority is immediately converted into triglycerides, which are sent out from the liver to be stored as fat in the adipose cells.[10]

If any one of the three components of that cycle worsens, the whole system worsens.

- If insulin resistance worsens, fat cells increase leptin secretion, which leads to leptin resistance, which further suppresses thyroid function.
- If leptin resistance worsens, thyroid suppression worsens, which results in worsening insulin resistance.
- If thyroid function drops, glucose metabolism is impaired, which worsens insulin resistance, which worsens leptin resistance.

Do you see the problem? It becomes a merry-go-round that spins faster and faster, but you can't get off it.

Now add in the fact that at least 40% of young adults in the US have insulin resistance. [11] Depending on the area of the country, the amount of all adults with insulin resistance exceeds 50%.

In my own practice, I found that about two-thirds of all people that we saw for corporate wellness visits met the criteria for either prediabetes or diabetes, all of which had insulin resistance.

There is less data available on the presence of leptin resistance. However, since leptin resistance is directly linked to obesity and this study showed that three-fourths of the US population is overweight or obese[12], it is safe to assume that the majority of people deal with some level of leptin resistance.

Finally, it is estimated that 23% of adults in the US are hypothyroid, which I believe is grossly underestimated.

So, in other words, most of us have some degree of insulin resistance and leptin resistance. Both are associated with being overweight or obese.

Now, add thyroid disease to that equation. With those three conditions at play, almost everyone will have weight issues.

So, what, if anything, can we do about it? That's the subject of the next chapter.

SUMMARY

- The "calorie in, calorie out" and "eat less, exercise more" concepts of weight loss simply don't work.

- Severe calorie-reduced diets over a period of time can severely damage your metabolism.

- The real cause of weight gain and obesity is an imbalance of your hormones, not an imbalance of your calories.

- Insulin resistance, leptin resistance, and thyroid conditions all affect each other and lead to worsening weight gain and weight loss resistance.

- A weight loss program that doesn't address those hormone issues will ultimately fail every single time.

11.

HOW TO LOSE WEIGHT IF YOU HAVE A THYROID CONDITION

"Paula" is a 52-year-old female who presented to my office. She complained of several symptoms affecting her quality of life—severe fatigue, weight gain, insomnia, night sweats, decreased libido, hair loss, and mood swings.

She felt fine until her mid-40s, when her menstrual cycle became extremely irregular and unpredictable. Her gynecologist performed a uterine ablation, which reduced her periods to a more manageable 1-3 days per month. However, her other symptoms continued to worsen. She gained about 20 pounds over the next few years, and her mood swings, night sweats, and fatigue continued to progress. By the time she came to my office, she had not had a menstrual cycle in almost two years. She had also begun to have several episodes of hot flashes throughout the day.

Her physical exam was unremarkable except for a weight of 142 pounds (she is 5'1").

Initial lab work showed a mildly elevated TSH of 2.78, a low free T3 of 2.6, normal reverse T3 of 10.3, negative thyroid antibodies, a total testosterone of 0, an estradiol of 0, a vitamin D of 22, a B12 of 527 and an FSH of 54.

She was treated with NDT Thyroid, adrenal adaptogens, vitamin D3 with K2, a methylated B vitamin, selenium, and nightly oral micronized progesterone. She was started on bioidentical testosterone and estradiol pellets, which she received subcutaneously every 3-4 months.

When she came back to the office a few months later, she stated that she felt better than she had in many years. She was sleeping well without sweating, her libido had improved, her mood had normalized, her hair loss had stopped, and she had started losing some weight. She had also started intermittent fasting 16 hours each day with a 2 or 3-day fast once or twice a month. She was staying active by keeping her young grandchildren during the week.

Two years after her first visit, her weight was down to 115 pounds, and she had maintained that weight for the past several months.

Hopefully, you now have a better understanding of why it is hard for you to lose weight if you have a thyroid condition.

So, what can you do? How can you reach the goal of having a successful, permanent weight loss?

These steps have been successful for my patients. This is not easy, but it is doable if you are motivated and disciplined.

Just like with most things, a half-hearted effort will result in half-hearted results. It is important to keep one thing in mind: Avoid thyroid "tunnel vision." There are likely several causes of your weight gain, not just your thyroid condition.

Of course, addressing your thyroid aggressively will make you feel better and improve your ability to lose weight.

However, changing or adding thyroid medication will, at most, lead to a 5 to 10-pound weight loss.

You are likely going to need to do several other things to get the weight off and keep it off.

1. INTERMITTENT FASTING IS IMPORTANT

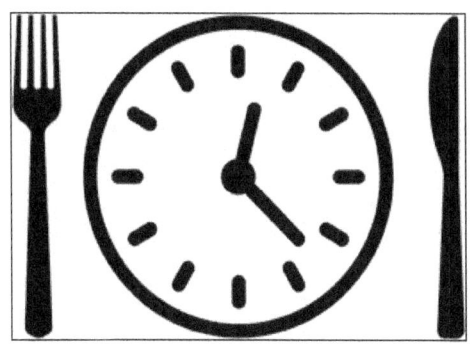

As I stated in the previous chapter, weight gain is an issue of hormone imbalances, NOT calorie imbalances.

The only way to have successful, long-term weight loss is to rebalance your hormones—primarily insulin, leptin, cortisol, and thyroid.

So, how do we balance those hormones? Let's start with insulin and leptin first.

The only way to permanently resolve insulin resistance and leptin resistance is to reduce the levels of those hormones long enough to allow the cells to "re-sensitize" to them.

Anything that reduces your intake of sugar and carbs will result in less insulin being secreted in the body.

No diet will do this as well as not eating anything at all.

Yes, fasting is by far the most potent tool we have to reduce insulin resistance (and ultimately leptin resistance). This fact has been known for centuries but has been scientifically confirmed.

Extensive research has been done over the past 70 years about the benefits of fasting as a treatment for various conditions, including obesity, type 2 diabetes, dementia, and even cancer.

Now, wait a minute. If severe low-calorie diets damage your metabolism (see Chapter 10), wouldn't fasting do the same thing?

The answer is a definite no.

When used correctly, intermittent fasting can actually repair your metabolism, not damage it.

The human body will adjust to a constant low-calorie diet by reducing the number of calories it burns (our metabolic rate).

Our body is designed to maintain the "status quo," including our weight (even when our weight is excessive).

For example, if your ideal body weight is 150 pounds, but you have weighed 175 pounds for the past few years, your body now thinks you should weigh 175 pounds.

If you reduce your calorie intake and start exercising, you can probably lose 10-15 pounds fairly quickly. However, your body thinks you should weigh 175, so your leptin and ghrelin secretion changes. Your hunger increases, and your metabolism drops.

That is why you invariably level off on your weight loss and eventually gain it back within a few weeks.

The opposite is true as well.

If you start eating more than usual and/or reduce your physical activity, your body realizes it is gaining weight. It will adjust the leptin and ghrelin secretion so that your appetite will decrease and your metabolism will increase in an attempt to get you back to your "normal" weight of 175 pounds.

When you eat a prolonged, severe, low-calorie diet, your body will eventually adjust to that diet by increasing your hunger and lowering your metabolism.

Remember, your body is trying to maintain your current weight. You basically stay "locked" in starvation mode.

Since intermittent fasting is done *intermittently,* the body never has a chance to make that adjustment.

As a result, the metabolism isn't reduced. If anything, it increases.

When intermittent fasting is utilized correctly, the cells become more sensitized to insulin and leptin. In effect, they start responding to those two hormones more efficiently.

This results in your "weight thermostat" dropping to a number closer to your desired weight. The longer you incorporate the fasting, the lower the thermostat number will be set.

Let's use the example from earlier.

Let's say you weigh 175 pounds, but you want to weigh 150 pounds. After incorporating some intermittent fasting for a few weeks, you drop some weight (maybe to 165 pounds), your body now considers

165 pounds to be where you should be because it has begun to re-sensitized itself to insulin and leptin.

If you continue the fasting program, what your body thinks is your "normal" body weight will continue to drop until you eventually reach your goal weight of 150 (assuming that is a reasonable weight for you and not an unrealistic weight).

There are several ways to do intermittent fasting. You may need to try various ones to see which your body responds to the best.

- **Daily 16-hour Fast** - Only eat in an 8-hour time period each day. For example, skip breakfast daily. This diet works best when you combine it with a low-carb diet. Weight loss occurs, but it is slow and gradual.
- **Daily 20-hour Fast** - Also called The Warrior Diet. This was popularized by Ori Hofmekler in the early 2000s. It was inspired by ancient warrior tribes such as the Spartans, who typically battled all day and then would feast in the evenings. This diet works best with a whole-food diet and regular high-intensity interval training.[1]
- **24-hour Fast** - Eating is limited to only once per day. You can fast from morning to morning, evening to evening, or mid-day to mid-day. This diet is helpful if you are on medication that should be taken with food (iron, aspirin, etc.). This fast was popularized by Brad Pilon in "Eat, Stop, Eat." He recommends doing two 24-hour fasts per week. In our experience, doing the two 24-hour fasts on consecutive days is particularly effective at losing weight. We recommend doing

a 16-hour fast on the other days of the week. This fast is particularly effective at reducing insulin resistance and stimulating weight loss.[2]

- **The 5:2 Diet** - This is really not a fast, but is a great starting point for anyone who is hesitant to try fasting. It consists of five normal eating days. On the other two days, women can eat up to 500 calories, and men may eat up to 600 calories. The fasting days can either be done consecutively or split up during the week. The calories can either be eaten in one meal on the fasting days or spread out over the day. If weight loss is not occurring as fast as you would like, you can then transition to a more strict fasting plan.[3]

- **Alternate-Day Fasting** - If you like the 5:2 diet but need a bit more aggressive approach, this is a good option. Just as in the 5:2 diet, during the "fasting" days, women can eat 500 calories, and men can eat 600 calories. However, the "fasting" days occur every other day, so there are actually 3-4 "fasting" days per week instead of just two. Several studies have shown this diet to be effective at weight loss.[4]

- **36-hour Fast** - This is the diet of choice for Dr. Jason Fung and his Intensive Dietary Management (IDM) program. With this diet, you don't eat for an entire day; then you don't eat until breakfast the next day. This fast is recommended 2-3 days per week. This is an excellent diet for anyone with severe insulin resistance (including prediabetes and type 2 diabetes). If you are diabetic, do NOT try this diet without involving your medical provider and closely monitoring your blood glucose.[5]

- **Longer Fasts** - Several experts, including Dr. Fung, routinely start patients with severe type 2 diabetes on 7 to 14-day fasts. They typically see a rapid improvement in insulin resistance with only rare medical complications. Oncologists have also started recommending yearly 7-day fasts for cancer patients due to their success in lowering cancer risk. If you want to consider a prolonged fast, please consult with your medical provider first to ensure your safety. It will be important to drink extra water and even consume a teaspoon of table salt daily to help prevent electrolyte imbalances. Consuming bone broth is also helpful.

- I don't recommend fasting in pregnant or breastfeeding women, children under the age of 18, or someone who is already underweight or malnourished. If you have gout, type 1 diabetes, or take prescription medication, consult with your medical provider before attempting any fast.

Keep in mind, the more severe the hormone imbalance and the longer you have had the imbalance, the longer it will take to reverse the insulin and leptin resistance. It can take months or even longer in some cases.

2. LOOK AT OTHER HORMONES BESIDES THYROID

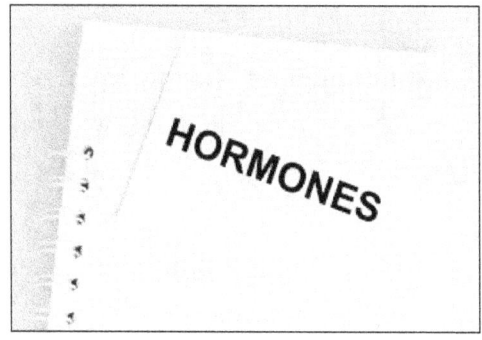

- **Insulin** - I discussed both insulin and leptin in detail in Chapter 10. Basically, if you are having weight issues, you undoubtedly have some level of insulin resistance.

This can be evaluated by getting a fasting glucose, hemoglobin A1c, and fasting insulin. A fasting glucose >100, a hemoglobin A1c >5.6, and a fasting insulin >5 are all indicators of insulin resistance and prediabetes or even diabetes.

The insulin resistance must be addressed, or nothing else we are discussing will result in long-lasting results.

Insulin resistance can mostly be improved with lifestyle changes. Low sugar, low simple carb, whole food diets are a necessity. Intermittent fasting is a must. Regular activity/exercise is helpful. Stress reduction is very important.

There are various supplements that can be of benefit as well. These include chromium, alpha lipoic acid, and berberine.

In severe cases, medication may be required at least for a period of time. We discuss a few of those later in this chapter.

- **Leptin** - Just like insulin resistance, leptin resistance is present in essentially everyone who is overweight or struggling to lose weight.

The interaction between insulin, leptin, thyroid, and cortisol has been well described in medical studies.

When excess fat is present in the body, it is likely that the hypothalamus has stopped responding to the chronically high leptin levels that were secreted by fat cells.

Re-sensitizing the body to leptin is a critical step in losing weight and keeping it off.

Periodically evaluating a serum leptin level can give you information on the severity of your leptin resistance and its response to your treatment plan.

All of the information that pertains to other hormone issues discussed in this chapter should also help reverse leptin resistance.

- **Testosterone** - Many of the symptoms of testosterone issues are the same as symptoms of thyroid deficiency. These include fatigue, weight gain, insomnia, cold intolerance, mood swings, brain fog, and others.

Clinically, it can be very hard to tell them apart based on symptoms alone.

There is a reason for that.

The hormonal systems of the body are very much intertwined with each other. If one system is dysfunctional, it tends to cause dysfunction in other systems.

That is definitely true for thyroid and testosterone.

Hypothyroidism has been shown to suppress testosterone production.[6, 7] If you are at all curious why, here is what happens:

Researchers have observed a chain reaction that can take place starting in the thyroid gland.

Proper production of thyroid hormone stimulates the hypothalamus, resulting in the production of GnRH (gonadotropin-releasing hormone).

GnRH then signals the pituitary gland to produce LH (luteinizing hormone). LH signals the testes to produce testosterone.

If this system starts off with poor production of thyroid hormone (hypothyroidism), a normal level of GnRH won't be produced, and the pituitary gland then won't get the proper message, causing low production of LH. Poor LH production means the testes won't be signaled to produce enough testosterone.

Hypothyroidism can also cause an increase in prolactin levels, a hormone that stimulates milk production in nursing mothers. Increased prolactin levels can also lower testosterone levels.[8]

The final result? You can be left with low testosterone levels.

That is why men and women with hypothyroidism tend to have low testosterone levels.

However, when thyroid hormone levels are normalized, testosterone levels often return to normal as well.

Of note, testosterone replacement can also significantly lower leptin levels.[9]

I often recommend normalizing thyroid levels before considering testosterone replacement therapy unless the testosterone levels are severely low and the patient is having debilitating symptoms.

Otherwise, if it doesn't return to normal or if the patient continues to have symptoms of low testosterone, I will then recommend treatment for the low testosterone.

Testosterone can be replaced in men via creams, gels, injections, or subcutaneous pellets. In women, I recommend either compounded creams or subcutaneous pellets.

Obviously, using a medical provider who is knowledgeable in testosterone replacement is critical.

In men, if your total testosterone level is <200, I recommend further workup, which would include a serum prolactin level and possible MRI imaging to rule out any pituitary issues.

- **Estrogen and Progesterone** - Most patients are diagnosed with thyroid issues in their 40s and 50s. When you think about the various hormone interactions, it makes sense.

As women enter the perimenopausal period, their ovaries stop producing a consistent amount of hormones every month.

Typically, progesterone levels start dropping a few years before estrogen levels drop. This can cause the menstrual cycles to become irregular and even unpredictable.

As estrogen levels maintain their normal levels (or close to it) and progesterone levels drop, the result is what we call estrogen dominance.[10]

As a general rule, a normal estrogen/progesterone ratio should be less than 100 to 1. When it gets more than that, the hormone system becomes imbalanced, resulting in things such as abnormal periods, water retention, breast tenderness, weight gain, mood swings, brain fog, fatigue, hair loss, and others.

Wait a minute, a lot of those symptoms sound like hypothyroidism, don't they?

That's because there is a good chance that the sex hormone imbalance is also impairing normal thyroid function (or vice-versa).

Progesterone and thyroid hormones are intimately connected. Progesterone improves the signaling mechanisms and also stimulates the production of TPO, the enzyme involved in making thyroid hormones.[11, 12]

Too little progesterone depresses TPO activity, lowering the production of thyroid hormones.

The estrogen dominance also increases liver production of sex hormone binding globulin (SHBG), which reduces the amount of free testosterone and free thyroid hormones.

This results in a situation where both sex hormone imbalance and thyroid dysfunction are occurring at the same time.

By the way, the same scenario can occur in someone taking oral contraceptive pills or hormone replacement therapy such as estradiol, Premarin, or Prempro.

These medications elevate the estrogen levels in the body even if progesterone levels are in the normal range. Elevated estrogen levels compared to progesterone levels (estrogen dominance) is still the result.

Depending on each individual situation, several things can be done.

Using micronized progesterone 100-400 mg daily at bedtime can help bring the excess estrogen back into balance. If you are still having a menstrual cycle, then progesterone is often prescribed nightly on days 15-28 of each cycle.

Obviously, stopping the oral contractive pill or hormone replacement pill can greatly reduce estrogen levels.

Even liver detoxification can help rebalance the hormones if estrogen levels are high and progesterone levels are normal.

All of this will require the help of your medical provider.

- **Cortisol** - Cortisol is our "stress hormone." When its levels are elevated, it signals the mitochondria in our cells to increase energy production to help us get through whatever stress is occurring.

When the body is functioning correctly, the cortisol will only be elevated for a short period of time, and then it will drop back to normal pre-stress levels.

Under high-stress situations such as chronic illness, serious injury, relationship issues, death in the family, working at a job you hate, etc., the cortisol level remains high for an extended period of time.

Studies have shown a definite link between cortisol levels and thyroid function.[13] The higher the cortisol level, the lower the thyroid function.

In fact, cortisol appears to have a direct effect on TSH secretion in the pituitary gland.
(14) In other words, cortisol directly suppresses thyroid function.

The link is so strong that we basically assume that any patient with a thyroid problem is also having adrenal/cortisol issues. When doing initial lab work on patients, checking their morning cortisol is a quick and easy way to quickly screen for any significant cortisol issues.

If the morning cortisol level is 10-20 micrograms/dL, it doesn't really tell us anything.

But if the morning cortisol is <10 or >20, it indicates there is likely an adrenal issue that needs to be further evaluated and treated. At that point, we typically order a DUTCH spot urine cortisol test, which will definitely evaluate cortisol levels. Salivary cortisol testing can be helpful as well.

Most hypothyroid patients will benefit from taking adrenal adaptogens. Those with a cortisol <10 should also consider taking adrenal glandulars for at least a few months until it increases to >10.

Learning some stress management techniques (yoga, meditation, and proper sleep hygiene) is a long-term solution to help lower cortisol levels, keep them low, and allow healthy weight loss to occur.

3. FOCUS ON THE QUALITY OF YOUR FOOD, NOT THE CALORIES

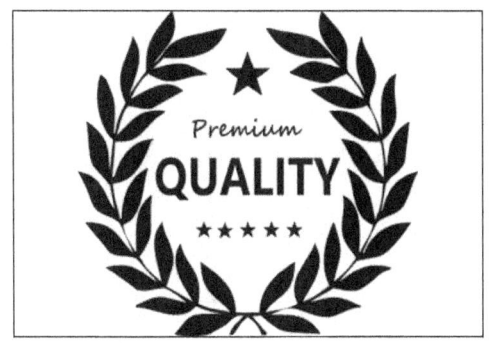

When you do eat, it's more important to control WHAT you eat than HOW MUCH you eat.

Obsessing over calories just doesn't work. Counting calories to lose weight has a 99% failure rate.

The failure rate is even higher in thyroid patients.

To make matters worse, calorie restriction makes thyroid function worse.

Sustained calorie restriction lowers T3[15], raises reverse T3[16], and lowers metabolism.[17]

One study even found that after just four weeks of a very low-calorie diet (400 calories per day), it dropped T3 levels by as much as 66%.[18]

In the same study, even a less severe calorie diet of 1000 calories per day reduced T3 levels by as much as 22%.

Even after you return to a normal diet, the damage to thyroid function continues for a long time.

So, if reducing calories is bad (especially if you have a thyroid condition), what can you do instead?

Start by focusing on eating good quality, whole food instead of low-calorie processed food. Just because something is low in calories doesn't mean it is good for you or will help you lose weight.

I like to tell people to eat "God food."

Ask yourself, "Did God make this, or did man make this?" If the answer is manmade, avoid it. That means it is processed and likely full of ingredients that will impair or even prevent weight loss, even if it is low in calories.

"Low calorie" is a marketing ploy. Don't fall for it.

Even if you lose weight initially when eating these foods, the weight will always come back because of metabolic adaptation and hormone imbalances that we discussed previously.

4. LEARN TO COOK

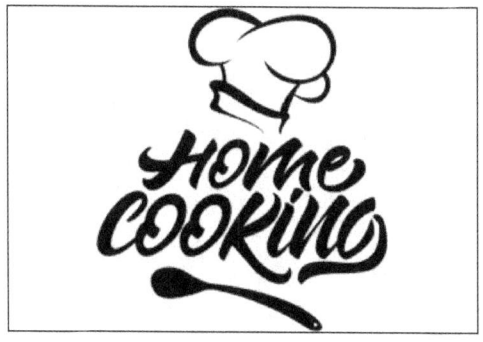

If you don't learn to cook and start making home-cooked meals the primary source of nutrition in your home, you will probably never lose weight or have sustained weight loss.

It really is that simple.

Learning to cook is the skill that allows you to transform boring, healthy foods into something that tastes delicious.

If you try to eat food that is good for you but doesn't necessarily taste good, you will eventually reject that food as a regular part of your diet.

But if something tastes delicious, you are more likely to eat it on a consistent basis and get the results you are looking to achieve.

It's hard enough as it is to transition from a diet full of processed foods to one that contains whole, healthy foods. Making healthy food taste good is a must for long-term success.

Why does processed food taste so good? It is totally by design.

Researchers have studied food immensely and know what makes it irresistible.[19] This includes things such as the texture of the food[20] and adding extra salt and sugar.[21]

This transition to whole food may be harder than you think. At first, whole food may taste dull or bland.

But it does get better.

After a few weeks, your taste buds adjust[22], and you will find that whole foods have much more flavor than you originally thought.

However, getting to that 2 to 4-week point will be very difficult if you don't learn how to cook things to their ultimate potential in taste.

Let's take eggs as an example.

You can poach, fry, hard boil, scramble, and soft boil an egg. A skilled cook can prepare an egg in at least these five different ways[23] and make them all taste amazing.

Each variation has a different texture and flavor profile and brings variety to the same food, making it easier to consume consistently.

This same principle can be applied to just about any real food.

It won't be necessary to memorize hundreds of recipes as long as you master a few basic principles of cooking.

Doing this will allow you to stay on track and make dishes that you look forward to eating time and again.

There is a ton of cooking information available in places such as YouTube and various cooking channels. You can also look for cooking classes at your local community college.

5. GETTING HEALTHIER IS MORE IMPORTANT THAN GETTING THINNER

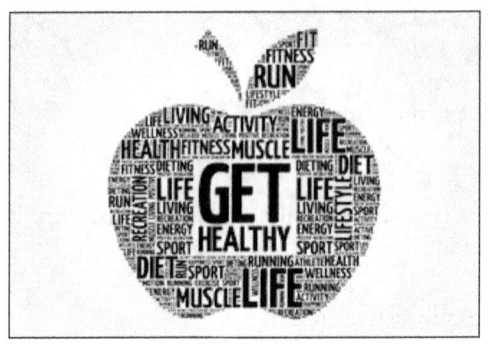

Society teaches us that being thin is healthy. That isn't always true. While it is true that being overweight or obese is unhealthy, losing weight doesn't automatically make you healthy.

It is quite possible to lose weight in the wrong way. In fact, it can actually make you more unhealthy and will lead to more weight gain in the future.

We have seen multiple patients who lost weight by crash dieting or other unhealthy techniques. The resulting nutrient deficiencies and hormone imbalances led to worsening fatigue, hair loss, menstrual irregularities, skin problems, and other issues.

Do those symptoms sound like someone who is healthy? Not even close. Those types of diets lead to both fat loss AND muscle loss. Instead, your goal should be to lose fat mass while preserving your lean muscle mass.[24]

So, what does getting healthier really mean?

It includes:

- Eating real whole foods
- Replacing nutrient deficiencies
- Managing stress
- Getting enough sleep
- Regular exercise
- Intermittent fasting

Each one of these topics deserves its own book. For now, we will leave it to you to pursue each one and find what works for you.

Keep in mind that a healthy weight loss program will not be fast. "Slow and steady" wins the race.

Approximately 5-10 pounds of weight loss per month should be your goal. Remember, this journey is a marathon, not a sprint.

6. EXERCISE IS IMPORTANT

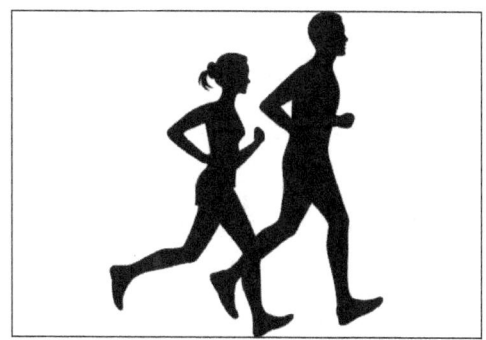

Have you ever heard someone say, "You can't out-exercise a bad diet?"

That is a fact.

As I discussed in the previous chapter, the "eat less, exercise more" theory of weight loss has been proven wrong over and over again, especially for thyroid patients.

Over-exercising damages the thyroid, increases cortisol, and may even impair your sex hormones.

It is not uncommon for extreme female athletes to stop having a menstrual cycle altogether due to their diet and exercise routines.[25]

Some experts estimate that exercise accounts for less than 10% of any healthy weight loss.

Still, there is no doubt that incorporating regular, healthy exercise will improve your overall health, maintain lean muscle mass, and will make an impact on your ability to lose weight.

So, what is a good exercise program to consider? Here are our suggestions:

- **Daily low-intensity exercise** - No matter what other types of exercise you choose to do throughout the week, you should always supplement them with

- daily low-intensity activity. This could include walking, light jogging, swimming, biking, or even just working around your house. Staying active throughout the day should be a priority. This should be done in addition to the other exercises we recommend.

- **Weekly strength training** - Strength training helps build muscle mass, which can improve metabolism and thyroid function. This is a necessity for anyone trying to lose weight, especially thyroid patients. Strength training should be limited to no more than 1-3 times per week.

- **Yoga** - Yoga is a great way to exercise, improve your flexibility, and reduce your stress. It can enhance your breathing and improve thyroid function.[26] It is critical for high stress people. We typically recommend yoga 1-3 times per week.

- **Periodic high-intensity interval training** - It is very important to add some high-intensity interval training (HIIT). This includes exercises that get your heart rate up to 70% of your maximal heart rate (calculate this by subtracting your age from 220 and then multiplying by 0.7). This type of exercise requires a lot of energy expenditure and will leave you breathless. You can certainly get this by joining an aerobics or cycling class at a local gym. You can also do HIIT training with just about any exercise machine or even with walking/running. For example, exercise hard (or run) for 30 seconds, then slow your pace to a casual pace for another 30 seconds to a minute. If you repeat the process 8-10 times, you have completed 15-20 minutes of HIIT training. The variation in heart rate is believed to be what stimulates your metabolism to increase.

- Keep in mind that if your exercise exhausts you for the rest of the day, you are either overdoing it or you could have some adrenal issues. Good, healthy exercise may initially exhaust you, but that should be followed by a feeling of relaxation, energy, and maybe even mild euphoria. If that isn't you, discuss it with your medical provider to make sure it is safe for you to continue.

7. SUPPLEMENTS CAN HELP

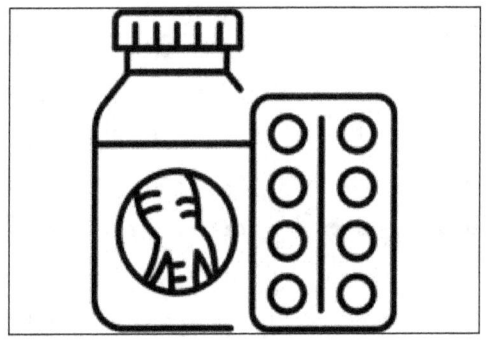

Let's put this out there from the start: The answer to your weight loss does not lie in which assortment of supplements you take.

You could take every single supplement in the list below and still not reach your weight loss goals, especially if you do nothing else that we mention in this chapter.

However, proper supplementation can indeed make an impact on the various imbalances that are causing your weight gain and/or weight loss resistance.

Depending on your current situation, some of these supplements may help more than others.

I broke these down by hormone imbalance to help you decide which you should consider.

- **Leptin-lowering supplements** - This list isn't very long. As I have stated previously, leptin resistance is rarely found by itself. It is commonly associated with insulin resistance, thyroid issues, and adrenal issues.

Typically, it is better to focus on supplements targeted towards other hormone imbalances. However, there are some specific supplements that have been shown to lower leptin levels.

a. Glucosamine - Glucosamine reduces leptin levels and pain in osteoarthritis.[27] Typical dose is 1,500 mg daily.

b. Zinc - Zinc lowered by leptin and insulin resistance in a study in obese women.[28] Typical dose is 30-60 mg daily.

c. Oralvisc - Oralvis has been shown to help reduce leptin and other inflammatory cytokines in patients with osteoarthritis. I would not recommend taking this for the sole purpose of lowering your leptin level. However, combining it with glucosamine could help if you are having issues with osteoarthritis that are made worse by your excess weight.[29]

- **Insulin resistance and leptin resistance** - These supplements are designed to reduce insulin levels and/or reduce insulin resistance.

a. Berberine - Helps lower blood sugar levels by sensitizing the body to insulin and by lowering inflammation.[30] Doses as high as 2,000 mg per day may be needed to see results.

b. Chromium - Helps sensitize cells to insulin.[31] Consider using up to 1,000 mcg per day.

c. Alpha Lipoic acid - May improve peripheral neuropathy and is helpful in lowering both glucose and leptin levels.[32] Doses as high as 600 mg per day in sustained-release capsules tend to provide the best results.

d. Myoinositol - This powerful sugar alcohol directly helps lower both insulin and leptin.[33] To get the full benefit, consider taking at least 1,500 mg daily for six months.

- **Thyroid resistance and leptin resistance** - Much like insulin resistance, it is rare to see a patient with leptin resistance who doesn't also have thyroid resistance.

In thyroid resistance, the blood levels of thyroid hormones may be "normal," but cellular levels are low, as evidenced by low free T3 and/or high levels of reverse T3.

This often is associated with a LOW TSH, which can make medical providers and patients falsely believe that thyroid function is too high.

This results in a weight increase, increased leptin levels, and decreased thyroid hormone activity.

One of the best ways to treat this is to increase the conversion of T4 to T3. This will result in a decrease of T4 to reverse T3.

The following supplements can help:

   a. Zinc - Helps promote T4 to T3 conversion. Also acts as an anti-inflammatory agent and an antioxidant. Consider taking 30-60 mg per day.

   b. Selenium - Helps promote T4 to T3 conversion. It may also help in reducing autoimmunity and inflammation in patients with Hashimoto's. Typical dose is 200-400 mcg daily.

   c. Iron - Iron is required for proper thyroid cellular function. Low symptoms mimic hypothyroidism. Be careful not to take too much, which can cause symptoms such as nausea and constipation.

- **High cortisol and high leptin** - Studies show that as cortisol levels increase, the production and secretion of leptin increases as well.34

This means that ignoring high cortisol levels will make losing weight almost impossible.

If your morning cortisol level is >18, consider using these supplements:

   a. Phosphatidylserine - Doses as high as 800 mg taken daily have been shown to attenuate cortisol levels.[35] Any levels >30 should be evaluated for possible Cushing's.

   b. Adrenal adaptogens - These may help balance adrenal function and lower cortisol levels.[36] They may also help improve energy levels and promote normal sleep patterns. Typical dose is two capsules every morning.

- **Improve sleep and lower leptin** - Lack of sleep is a huge reason that patients develop and get worsening leptin resistance.

This is so important that if you do everything we have discussed but continue to get inadequate sleep, you will not resolve your leptin resistance.

Lack of sleep has been shown to alter blood sugar homeostasis and lead to weight gain.[37, 38]

Getting eight hours of uninterrupted sleep is a necessity for any successful weight loss program.

Even if you feel like you can function on less sleep, it may still be destroying your body from a metabolic standpoint.

Supplements that can improve the depth and quality of sleep are listed below from least aggressive to most aggressive:

a. 5-HTP - This is a gentle way to promote healthy sleep, especially when it is due to mood-related issues. Start with 100 mg taken 30 minutes before bedtime, which can be increased to 200 mg if needed.

b. Melatonin - Melatonin can help promote regular circadian rhythm. It is especially helpful for people who travel to different time zones or who work varying time shifts. Start with 1-3 mg nightly and increase as needed.

c. GABA + serotonin potentiators - These act by enhancing the effects of both serotonin and GABA neurotransmitters. They can help slow down the brain and induce delta wave production to increase the depth of sleep. Frequently used with melatonin. Typical dose is one capsule per night.

8. PRESCRIPTION MEDS THAT CAN HELP

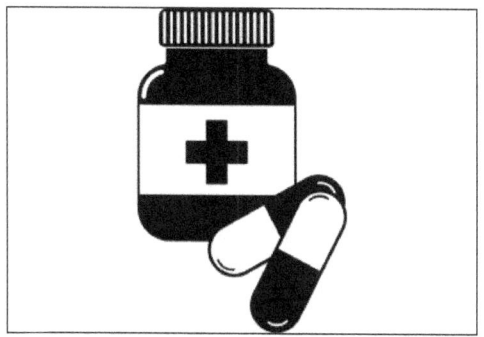

Most weight loss medications target your appetite and attempt to reduce the number of calories you are consuming.

Hopefully, you understand by this point in the book that reducing calories helps with weight loss for only a short period of time, if at all. Eventually, 99% of calorie counters will gain their weight back.

Instead of focusing on appetite, you need to focus on balancing leptin levels, optimizing thyroid function, and reducing insulin resistance.

Below are some prescription medications that have been shown in studies to result in long-term weight loss.

These must be written by a medical provider (doctor, PA, or NP).

- **GLP-1 Agonists** - Glucagon-like peptide agonists are FDA-approved to treat type 2 diabetes. However, they also reduce leptin resistance.

Two of these medications, Saxenda and Wegovy, are actually FDA-approved for weight loss, but the others are not.

They were created to treat type 2 diabetes but were later found to have a profound effect on weight.

They reduce appetite, but they also improve leptin sensitivity and insulin sensitivity.[39]

They stimulate insulin secretion in the hyperglycemic state.

They suppress glucagon secretion in the hyperglycemic and euglycemic state.

They also delay gastric emptying, which results in a decrease in appetite and the sensation of feeling full sooner when eating.

GLP-1 agonists also help prevent the drop in leptin that occurs after a period of weight loss.[40]

More recent studies also show a reduction in major adverse cardiac events, reduced neural degeneration, reduced blood pressure, and a reduction in inflammation.

There appears to be an increased risk for pancreatitis and certain types of thyroid cancer.

Another concern is the potential for loss of lean muscle mass. Any patient that is taking a GLP-1 agonist MUST be on a regular weight-training regimen.

Unfortunately, GLP-1 agonists are extremely expensive, and insurance will typically not pay for them for any diagnosis other than type 2 diabetes.

There are coupons that can be used to offset the cost, and your medical provider can be creative with their coding if they are willing to work with you.

Dosages vary with each medication. As a general rule, I recommend starting on the lowest dose. If there is no response in 2-3 months, then increase the dose if you can tolerate it.

Examples of GLP-1 agonist medications:

1. Byetta
2. Bydureon
3. Victoza
4. Trulicity
5. Ozempic
6. Wegovy
7. Adlyxin
8. Rybelsus
9. Saxenda

- **Metformin** - Metformin has been around for many years. Although used primarily for the treatment of type 2 diabetes, it also has many other off-label uses. These include PCOS, early insulin resistance, anti-cancer, and even anti-aging.[41]

Relative to this discussion, it appears to have some impact on reducing leptin levels.[42]

This decrease in leptin is very helpful if you have leptin resistance and need to lower your leptin level temporarily to help promote leptin sensitivity.[43]

The good news about metformin is it is inexpensive, and medical providers are more likely to write a prescription for it than some of the other meds, such as GLP-1 agonists.

The bad news is it just isn't very powerful for treating leptin resistance and lowering weight. One study showed an average weight loss of 10-15 pounds when taking up to 2500 mg of metformin.[44]

If you have mild leptin resistance, metformin should be a consideration. If you have moderate or severe leptin resistance, it is largely ineffective.

Metformin is almost never given as a standalone weight-loss medication. However, it can be used in conjunction with other medications and treatments with some added benefit.

Metformin is notorious for causing GI side effects—mainly nausea and diarrhea. This often improves over time, or there is an extended-release version that helps, although it is much more expensive.

Typical dose is 500 mg to 2500 mg daily.

- **Naltrexone** - Naltrexone was originally developed as a treatment for opioid and alcohol dependence. It has also gained popularity in recent years as a treatment for autoimmune conditions. I have had great success using it as a treatment for Hashimoto's thyroiditis, where it appears to modulate the immune system and help lower autoantibodies.[45]

Recently, naltrexone has received FDA approval for weight loss when it is combined with Wellbutrin. The brand name is called Contrave.

Although I rarely use the combination drug due to cost, naltrexone by itself can lead to weight loss.[46]

In my experience, it is a safe medication. The worst side effect that I see with it is vivid dreams when taking higher doses.

The lower dosages are not available in standard pharmacies. You will need to have your medical provider order it from a compounding pharmacy.

If you are currently taking an opioid medication for pain, then naltrexone is contraindicated. It will block the effects of the opioid medication, which could cause an acute pain reaction.

Otherwise, this medication is a great option for people with an autoimmune condition such as Hashimoto's thyroiditis and who are struggling to lose weight.

I typically start with 1.5-3 mg at bedtime, then increase it by 1.5 mg every few weeks as needed to a maximum dose of around 9 mg.

- **SGLT-2 Inhibitors** - These medications are FDA approved for treating type 2 diabetes, but they have also been shown to be effective in promoting weight loss.

They work by preventing your kidneys from absorbing sugar in your bloodstream. The net result is you eliminate the extra sugar in your urine.

SGLT-2 inhibitors probably help reduce leptin resistance by directly impacting leptin sensitivity.

One study showed this drug downregulates leptin release, which helps improve leptin sensitivity.[47]

If you have type 2 diabetes or severe insulin resistance, it might be worth exploring this class of medication.

They appear to be effective for weight loss as well.[48]

In my experience, they are not as effective as GLP-1 agonists but are more effective than metformin.

Unfortunately, they are also extremely expensive.

The most common side effect I see is genital yeast infections. Yeast loves sugar, so spilling a lot of it in your urine can provide an environment where yeast can grow.

Medications in this class include:
- Invokana
- Farxiga
- Jardiance
- Steglatro
- Brenzavvy

- **Calcitonin** - Calcitonin is actually a hormone produced by your thyroid gland, and its primary job is to help maintain calcium levels.

But I'm not really interested in its ability to balance your calcium. I am more interested in the fact that calcitonin is also an amylin agonist.

An agonist simply refers to the fact that something stimulates or promotes a certain function. This can be compared to the word an-tagonist, which does the exact opposite.

So, in this setting, an amylin agonist is something that promotes the effects of amylin.

The question then becomes, what is amylin?

Amylin is a VERY important hormone secreted by the pancreas with insulin, which helps to balance blood sugar, balance your appetite, and alter how fast or slow you absorb foods.

Calcitonin may, therefore, indirectly act on amylin to promote those very functions.

This is why it can be used as an off-label medication to treat leptin resistance.

Much like the other medications listed here, calcitonin is not FDA-approved for treating leptin levels.

Instead, it is often used to treat osteoporosis because of its effects on calcium regulation.

For the purposes of this book, I don't care about that component, but I do care about the fact that it acts as an amylin agonist.[49]

Calcitonin can be used as a medication in the form of salmon calcitonin.

Salmon calcitonin, derived from salmon (the fish), is similar to human calcitonin but not the exact same.[50]

In fact, salmon calcitonin is about 40-50 times more powerful than human calcitonin.[51]

There have been some concerns over the side effects of salmon calcitonin, like the other medications listed here, but I don't think these side effects are a big concern.

Why?

Because your only purpose in using these medications is to reverse your leptin levels and help you lose weight.

Once you reverse this condition, you can stop using the medication.

This means that you really won't be on any of these medications long-term.

I think it could be argued that staying 30-50 pounds overweight for 20-30 years is FAR more likely to cause harm to your body than the temporary use of these medications.

We know that obesity definitely increases your risk of heart disease, stroke, diabetes, metabolic syndrome, cancer, and other serious conditions.[52]

Most people absolutely trade long-term weight loss and a definite decrease in risk of heart disease and cancer for a short-term and possible risk of various side effects related to certain prescription medications.

Salmon calcitonin is used as a nasal spray and runs around $30-$40 per month, which makes it relatively affordable compared to some of the other medications we have discussed.

9. CONSIDER THE REVERSE DIET IF YOU HAVE A DAMAGED METABOLISM

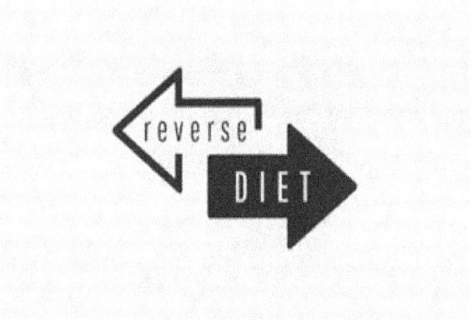

If you think that you have a damaged metabolism because of crash dieting and other activities in the past, there is hope.

People with metabolic damage tend to only get worse over time because they try to correct the problem by continuing to do the things that damaged their metabolism in the first place—namely, severe low-calorie dieting and excessive exercise.

The vicious cycle continues until some people are eating 1000 calories or less daily just to try to maintain their weight.

The reverse diet is a potential solution to this problem.[53] But it comes at a cost, which I will discuss.

How do you reverse diet?

Basically, you increase your daily calorie consumption by about 200 calories per day every few weeks until you are consuming what is considered a normal number of calories daily (about 1600 for women, about 2000 for men).

If you increase your calorie consumption consistently and for a period of time, your metabolism will gradually improve. This can take 3-6 months or longer, depending on your level of metabolic damage.

This ultimately results in an improvement in thyroid function, insulin resistance, and leptin resistance.[54]

But it will come at a temporary cost: a potential weight gain of 5-10 pounds (or even more).

If that seems unacceptable, there, unfortunately, aren't any other good options.

You could keep doing what you're doing and slowly starve yourself without any appreciable weight loss.

You could continue to cycle severe low-calorie diets and extreme exercise in exchange for minimal to no weight loss.

A temporary mild weight gain in exchange for an improved metabolism and a more balanced hormonal system is probably a good deal.

It is important to make sure you need this diet before trying it. Otherwise, you could potentially gain weight without getting any added benefit.

Potential candidates for the reverse diet include:
- People who have been unable to lose weight despite restricting their daily calories (1200 calories or less)
- People who don't respond to calorie-restricted diets like they used to.
- You suffer from constant low body temperature, low resting heart rate, low energy, and hair loss, especially if these symptoms occur after dieting.
- You have high reverse T3 levels, and low free T3 levels are dieting.
- You are already eating healthy and have tried various other healthy types of diets without success.

246

Only if you fit into one of these categories would I recommend considering a reverse diet.

10. CONSIDER ENVIRONMENTAL TOXINS AND DETOXIFICATION

There are several environmental toxins that have been shown to cause weight gain. They are called obesogens.

These toxins can contribute to weight gain by altering metabolism, hormone balance, and fat storage.[55] They can overwhelm our body's ability to detoxify itself, resulting in inflammation.

They can also disrupt the normal hormone signaling of the body. They can even alter our normal metabolism and promote the growth of fat cells.

Animal studies show that toxic chemicals can cause weight gain independent of any change in calorie intake or physical activity.

They can be found in things such as our food, water, perfume, cleaning products, makeup, and toiletries.

Some of the most common include:

1. Bisphenol-A (BPA) - BPA is the ultimate endocrine-disrupting chemical. The amount of BPA is directly correlated with the level of obesity in children in a recent study.[56] BPA is found in plastic storage containers, water bottles, and paper receipts.

2. Phthalates - Phthalates are commonly found in makeup, air fresheners, lotions, and various plastics. One study showed that exposure to BPA and phthalates leads to oxidative stress and insulin resistance in children.[57]

3. Perfluorinated Compounds (PFCs) - These chemicals are used almost everywhere because nothing sticks to them (can you say Teflon?). It can take more than four years for our body to break them down. They are known endocrine disruptors that lower thyroid function and alter sex hormones.[58]

4. Artificial sweeteners - These commonly used products can alter your gut microbiome, which can lead to several chronic diseases, including obesity. High fructose corn syrup also worsens leptin resistance.[59]

5. Heavy Metals - Lead, cadmium, and mercury have long been known to cause immune dysfunction and inflammation. They have also recently been linked to metabolic syndrome, which leads to insulin resistance and obesity.[60] They also inhibit normal thyroid function.[61]

So, what can you do about the toxins that are seemingly everywhere?

There are several relatively simple ways to detoxify your body and reduce your toxic load:

- Eat organic when possible.
- Be aware of toxic skin products
- Avoid eating big fish with large mercury content
- Drink lots of water and eat lots of fiber
- Eat 1-2 cups of cruciferous vegetables such as broccoli, kale and bok choy.
- Consider supplements that support detoxification—selenium, zinc, vitamin C, NAC, alpha-lipoic acid, and milk thistle.
- Exercise and sweat regularly with a near-infrared sauna
- Avoid using herbicides and pesticides
- Avoid using antibacterial products

If you are still struggling to lose weight after following all of these recommendations, it is probably time to seek the help of a functional medicine provider who is trained in managing resistant weight loss and hormonal imbalances.

SUMMARY

- Weight loss is a complex, multi-factorial issue that is made worse with thyroid conditions.
- Any successful weight loss program must focus on reducing insulin resistance, leptin resistance, sex hormone imbalances, cortisol issues, and thyroid issues to achieve successful, permanent weight loss.
- Intermittent fasting is an important component of any long-term weight loss program.

- Eating good quality whole foods that you learn to prepare yourself is essential.
- Exercise can be helpful, particularly high-intensity interval training, to re-sensitize your body to leptin and insulin.
- Targeted supplements tailored to your specific conditions can be very beneficial.
- When significant insulin resistance and leptin resistance are present, pharmaceuticals may be needed for at least a short period of time.
- If you have a damaged metabolism from severe low-calorie dieting, reverse dieting may be required to restore your metabolic rate back to a normal level.
- Consider environmental toxins and start utilizing some basic steps to reduce your toxic exposure and to help your body detoxify itself.

12.

HOW TO FIND A DOCTOR
WHO WILL HELP YOU

So, I have discussed all the various thyroid diseases that plague so many people. I have shown how most people are not managed well.

I have also laid out how the latest research and my personal experiences have helped me develop a better way of diagnosing, treating, and managing people with thyroid problems.

Now that you have all this information, how do you find a doctor that will help you? None of this information does any good if you don't have a medical provider that will work with you.

Unfortunately, the prevailing thought in conventional medicine is that thyroid disease is easily treated. Thyroid treatment is essentially the same for all patients. If you continue to experience symptoms despite following the treatment plan, something else besides thyroid problems must be the cause (depression, fibromyalgia, etc.).

That simply isn't true most of the time.

So, how do you find a doctor who will help you? Here are some attributes to look for:

1. Are they willing to listen to you and try something new? Our knowledge of the body is constantly changing, and we are learning new things on a daily basis. It is more important than ever for medical providers to be open to new treatments or therapies.

With just about any occupation, I have found that this scenario holds true: If someone presents to 100 experts in that field a new or different way of doing something than what is considered to be the standard way of doing it, about 90-95% of the people will immediately dismiss it. They either feel the way they have always done it works fine, or they think the presenter and his or her idea is "crazy," or they simply don't want to have to learn a completely different way of doing it.

Only about 5-10% will say, "Interesting. I need to learn more about that." That is a broad generalization, but I have noticed it in many fields (including medicine).

Your goal should be to try to find one of those 5-10% of doctors who are open to new ideas and treatments. If your current doctor isn't willing to work with you, you may need to keep looking.

By the way, it is not worth wasting your time trying to educate your physician on what you have read in this book—that approach will never work. Instead, spend your time and energy finding someone who will listen and work with you. It is important to realize that you shouldn't expect a doctor to do treatments or prescribe medications that they have no experience using.

If your doctor isn't comfortable doing many of the things I discussed in this book, that's okay. Keep seeing them for your non-thyroid issues. You just may need to find someone else to specifically take care of your thyroid.

2. Are they willing to order a complete thyroid panel?
Hopefully, I have convinced you by now that you need more than a TSH to truly assess and monitor your thyroid function.

The standard of care in conventional medicine is to simply use the TSH when screening for and managing thyroid disease.

The TSH by itself is simply inadequate.

You can miss the presence of autoimmune thyroid disease, T4 to T3 conversion issues, and the impact of nutrient deficiencies such as selenium, zinc, and iodine.

I recommend that the following labs should be considered the standard lab tests in thyroid patients:
- TSH
- Free T4
- Free T3
- Reverse T3
- TPO Antibodies
- Thyroglobulin Antibodies

These lab tests as a group are much better at evaluating true thyroid hormone function in the body compared to only checking a TSH. Make sure your doctor is comfortable ordering them AND interpreting them. Please review Chapter 2 for more information.

3. Are they willing to use thyroid medications other than levothyroxine?

As I discussed in Chapter 9, there are many different thyroid medications that can be used with success in patients.

These other medications include natural desiccated thyroid (NDT) such as Armour Thyroid, NP Thyroid, and Nature-Throid. There are also T3 medications such as Cytomel or liothyronine, and T4 medications such as Tyrosint. Compounding pharmacies can also compound thyroid medication containing T4, T3, or both.

Since many thyroid patients have issues with T4 to T3 conversion, giving them T4-only medication such as levothyroxine may not work for them.

Other individuals may not absorb levothyroxine as well as other medications in their digestive tract, so they may benefit from using a different medication.

A doctor's willingness to prescribe something other than levothyroxine may be the quickest way for you to gauge their thyroid knowledge and willingness to try new therapies.

4. Do they understand the importance of thyroid antibodies?
As I discussed in Chapter 5, the presence of thyroid antibodies indicates that you may have a condition called Hashimoto's thyroiditis (autoimmune thyroid disease).

If the thyroid antibodies are present, they will eventually damage and even destroy the thyroid gland, which will cause permanent hypothyroidism.

Most conventional doctors avoid ordering these tests because they have been taught that nothing can be done to reverse the condition anyway. Instead, they take a "wait and see" approach. They are taught to periodically monitor TSH levels and begin thyroid medication when enough damage to the thyroid from the antibodies has occurred to merit thyroid medication.

This is unfortunate for several reasons.

For starters, thyroid antibodies themselves cause problems beyond damage to the thyroid. They have been shown to increase the risk of developing certain cancers.[1]

Also there are also many lifestyle changes, supplements, and medications that can be effective in reducing thyroid antibody levels.

If caught early in the disease process, it is possible to reduce and even completely stop the damage to the thyroid gland caused by Hashimoto's.

Make sure you find a doctor who is willing to test for thyroid antibodies and is willing to explore different treatment options.

5. Do they understand that all patients are different?

This may sound obvious, but the current standard of care for thyroid disease is to treat everyone with levothyroxine.

Doctors don't manage most other conditions with a blanket treatment, so we shouldn't be doing it with thyroid disease, either.

This is where the art of medicine comes into play.

Each person is genetically unique and, therefore, requires different treatments, therapies, diet, medication, etc.

As an example, for people who have a history of medication reactions or reactions to fillers and dyes, levothyroxine may not be a good choice for them. Tirosint, which has fewer fillers, may be better tolerated.[2]

There may be other people who have issues with T4 to T3 conversion because of other medical conditions going on in their bodies. In those situations, adding T3 or changing to an NDT medication may make them feel much better.

Blanket recommendations should be made for your bed, not your body!

6. Do they understand the interactions of thyroid hormone with other hormone systems?

The hormone systems of the body are all intertwined and dependent on each other. A dysfunction in one of those systems will often lead to dysfunction in others.

Adrenal dysfunction can impair normal thyroid function. Insulin resistance can affect essentially all other hormones. Estrogen, progesterone, and testosterone affect thyroid function and vice versa. Leptin resistance suppresses thyroid function.

These are just a few examples.

When they are dysregulated, many of these other hormonal systems cause symptoms very similar to thyroid problems. That is why just treating someone's thyroid problem may not make them feel as good as they could or should.

It's important to have a doctor who evaluates ALL the hormone systems and sees the body as the complex organism that it is.

TIPS AND TRICKS TO HELP YOU FIND GOOD THYROID DOCTORS

Unsure where to start your search for a thyroid doctor?

Here are a few ideas:

- Call some local pharmacies (especially compounding pharmacies) and ask them for a list of doctors who prescribe NDT, liothyronine, and compounded thyroid medication.
- Contact local lab testing centers and ask for a list of doctors who order the tests in the complete thyroid panel.
- Contact integrative and functional medicine websites and organizations for a list of member doctors in your area.
- Use Facebook support groups for doctor references.
- Look for doctors who have training or certifications in hormone therapy, integrative medicine, anti-aging medicine, and functional medicine.
- Look for doctors who have written blog posts or books about thyroid management. Or even ones who reside in the Amarillo, Texas, area and whose last names rhyme with "Melchel."

SHOULD I SEE AN ENDOCRINOLOGIST?

I am asked that question a lot. There are obviously many brilliant endocrinologists in the world. I have nothing but respect for their knowledge and their desire to help people.

My frustration is with how most were trained in the management of thyroid and sex hormones. They typically don't focus on bioidentical hormone replacement, and they tend to evaluate and treat most thyroid patients the same way.

As I have already discussed, I strongly believe that this conventional approach is inadequate for most thyroid patients.

If you have "typical" hypothyroidism but are otherwise healthy, the conventional standard of care of using levothyroxine may work great for you. However, if that is your story, you probably aren't going to feel the need to read this book in the first place!

WHAT ABOUT FUNCTIONAL AND INTEGRATIVE DOCTORS?

I had excellent conventional training in medical school and residency.

As I began my medical practice, I saw how conventional hormone treatment did not help a lot of my patients, so I started pursuing dif-ferent ways of managing them. That led to hours upon hours of self-study, plus attending integrative and functional medicine conferenc-es and seminars. I am therefore very positive about the impact of integrative/functional medicine providers, especially with chronic diseases.

The difficulty lies in the fact that many of those doctors operate outside of the insurance model.

That means you will need to pay cash for office visits and sometimes even labs. This can get quite expensive in some situations. Although I feel it is worth it if you can afford it, I realize this could be a limitation for many people.

It is important to keep in mind that having integrative or functional medicine training does <u>not</u> guarantee that doctors are experts in hormone management.

Make sure you research their specific areas of expertise before spending a lot of money.

SUMMARY

- Finding a doctor who will listen to you and be open to non-conventional thyroid treatments is essential if you want to reach your maximum level of thyroid health.

- Your doctor needs to feel comfortable using various thyroid medications other than levothyroxine. These include Tirosint, natural desiccated thyroid (NDT), and Cytomel (liothyronine).

- To truly evaluate and monitor your thyroid function, your doctor needs to perform more than TSH and T4 lab tests. These include free T3, reverse T3, TPO antibodies, and thyroglobulin antibodies.

- Helpful resources for finding a good thyroid doctor include calling your local pharmacy, asking Facebook support groups, contacting function or integrative websites, and calling your laboratory testing center.

13.

HOW ABOUT A COMPROMISE?

Okay, I get it.

Everything I have taught you in this book may only make things more frustrating for many of you.

The more information you learn about your thyroid, the more it may potentially cause an even bigger disconnect between you and your medical provider.

I hear it all the time. "I know I need to have more thyroid labs checked, but my doctor won't order them. What should I do?"

"My doctor tells me my thyroid is good. If that is true, then why am I still having so many symptoms that seem like they are thyroid related?"

"She will only prescribe levothyroxine for me. She won't even consider trying a different medication."

By now, I have beaten this to death, but what I am recommending in this book goes against the current thyroid treatment paradigm.

The current thyroid paradigm simply states:
- TSH is the single best screening test for primary thyroid dysfunction for the vast majority of outpatient situations.
- T4 is converted to T3 as needed. Therefore, levothyroxine is the only thyroid medication that is needed.
- A normal thyroid state is present if the TSH is within its reference range.

Conventional medical training teaches your doctor that any thyroid testing and management should be evaluated only through this lens.

The result of this is there are now two different thyroid treatment camps, and those camps are growing farther and farther apart.

Both approaches have some merit, but each side is also guilty of taking it too far.

Conventional doctors can appear stubborn and unwieldy, refusing to entertain any ideas or recommendations that patients may have found after doing their own research (like this book).

On the alternative/integrative side, medical providers and patients can tread into unstudied territory that can include treatments that have never been proven to be effective or may even be dangerous.

This makes the conventional side dig their heels in even more, which pushes the alternative side to be even more aggressive with unproven and untested treatments.

And the cycle continues.

So, how do we get this situation into a reasonable middle ground?

A commentary paper released by the Thyroid UK organization is a great consideration.[1]

It proposes some commonsense treatment recommendations that allow a more comprehensive evaluation of the thyroid that is completely backed by research and avoids stepping into untested and potentially dangerous territory.

It includes the following recommendations:
1. Diagnosis must always include a patient's full medical history.
2. Diagnosis must include an evaluation of symptoms, which reflect tissue thyroid responses, and the patient's well-being.
3. Where symptoms indicative of thyroid disease are present, an ultrasound of the thyroid is advisable.
4. Symptomatic testing and case finding should include TSH, FT4, and FT3, arguably Reverse T3, TPO ab, and TG ab (only if TPO is negative and TSH is high).
5. To avoid false test results[4], thyroid hormone medication should not be taken until after blood is drawn.

6. Multiple symptoms typical of hypothyroidism, accompanied by low FT4 and FT3 levels, are strongly indicative of hypothyroidism[5]. Both FT4 and FT3 levels should be individually monitored and increased as needed to relieve symptoms of hypothyroidism without creating symptoms of hyperthyroidism.

7. Cortisol, Vitamin D, B12, and ferritin should be considered and also optimized for symptom relief.[5, 9]

Let's break down each bullet point to see why this might be a middle ground that both sides should consider:

1. Diagnosis must always include a patient's full medical history.

Since many of the hypothyroid symptoms are nonspecific, they may not be due to a thyroid issue.

That is where a complete medical history and a good quality physical exam are important.

It is not uncommon for me to see patients who are convinced they have a thyroid condition when, in fact, they have issues with perimenopause/menopause or even symptoms due to their extreme diets.

2. Diagnosis must include an evaluation of symptoms, which reflect tissue thyroid responses, and the patient's well-being.

This is an important point that is missed in the current thyroid treatment paradigm.

Just because someone's TSH level is in the normal range, it does not mean that their thyroid function is guaranteed to be normal.

Different tissues of the body have different sensitivities to thyroid hormones because of the presence or absence of deiodinases (see Chapter 1).

If we see a patient with normal lab work but they still feel terrible, more workup and evaluation needs to be done.

We need to treat individuals, not their lab results. Let's listen to them and their symptoms.

3. Where symptoms indicative of thyroid disease are present, an ultrasound of the thyroid is advisable.

Getting a thyroid ultrasound is rarely done in most medical practices.

That's unfortunate because it is a cheap and effective way to get a good look at the thyroid gland.

It has the potential to help identify physical abnormalities such as nodules, goiter, and inflammation.

Detecting something like Hashimoto's early can allow for early treatments that can slow and even reverse some of these conditions.

While I don't typically order a thyroid ultrasound on hypothyroid patients, it is reasonable to consider it.

When up to 90% of hypothyroid cases occur because of Hashimoto's thyroiditis, it only makes sense to at least get a one-time ultrasound.

4. Symptomatic testing and case finding should include TSH, free T4, free T3, arguably reverse T3, TPO antibodies, and thyroglobulin antibodies (only if TPO is negative and TSH is high).

If you have read this far in this book or read my thyroid blog articles, you should know by now that these are the lab tests that I recommend for most thyroid patients.

This would allow for the possibility of earlier diagnosis of conditions such as Hashimoto's, receptor issues, or T4 to T3 conversion issues.

As I mentioned in Chapter 1, I find it fascinating and a bit bewildering that the thyroid is the only hormone of the pituitary-controlled hormones where testing the free hormone levels is not considered standard of care.

Free T3 and free T4 levels should be checked (in addition to TSH) to assess thyroid function. I'm not sure why that is controversial.
While I still like to check reverse T3 levels, I can see why they list reverse T3 as "arguable."

Recommending TPO antibodies and excluding thyroglobulin antibodies is also understandable.

TPO antibodies are more closely associated with Hashimoto's and hypothyroidism compared to thyroglobulin antibodies.

Instead, it is reasonable only to check thyroglobulin antibodies if TPO antibodies are normal, but the TSH is elevated.

Again, I like to have all six tests run most of the time (at least initially). However, these recommendations are a reasonable middle ground, and hopefully, conventional doctors will be more willing to consider them.

Simply having free T3 levels checked would be a vast improvement from current treatment protocols.

5. To avoid false test results, thyroid hormone medication should not be taken until after blood is drawn.

Taking your thyroid medication near the time when your blood work is drawn basically makes the free hormone levels results useless.

The results will look higher than they actually are.

In my opinion, the most important information for you and your provider is to know what your free thyroid hormone levels are at their lowest point.

In this case, it would be right before you normally take your medication for the day.

6. Multiple symptoms typical of hypothyroidism, accompanied by low free T4 and free T3 levels, are strongly indicative of hypothyroidism. Both free T4 and free T3 levels should be individually monitored and increased as needed to relieve symptoms of hypothyroidism without creating symptoms of hyperthyroidism.

This recommendation is for those myriad of patients who have a normal TSH but still have symptoms of hypothyroidism.

It suggests that the presence of low free T3 and/or low free T4, in combination with hypothyroid symptoms, is strongly suggestive of hypothyroidism regardless of what the TSH level shows.

This is where conventional medical providers are going to have to step out of their TSH mindset if they want to solve the persistent hypothyroid symptoms that plague many thyroid patients.

The language subtly suggests that the free thyroid hormones play more of a role in regulating thyroid status in the body than does the TSH.

This is also where the alternative side can take it too far, so they must be cautious.

If you focus solely on the free thyroid hormones and ignore the TSH entirely, it's very easy to take too much thyroid hormone in an attempt to optimize your free thyroid hormone levels.

A nice compromise would be to monitor both the TSH and the free hormone levels while also monitoring for both hypothyroid and hyperthyroid symptoms.

7. Cortisol, vitamin D, B12, and ferritin should be considered and also optimized for symptom relief.

Essentially, all alternative thyroid medical providers know how important these other factors are because of how they indirectly influence thyroid function.

However, these are not things that are stressed in the conventional world.

Testing for these deficiencies is important because their presence could be a sign of early thyroid dysfunction, or even cause their own symptoms, which can be mistaken for thyroid issues.

All seven of these recommendations are backed by scientific studies.

When there are strong studies to back up each point, they are harder to be dismissed by a provider that doesn't currently manage thyroid patients the same way as the recommendations.

If you are a medical provider, I ask you to research the extensive bibliographies listed at the end of this commentary and at the end of this book.

If you are a thyroid patient who doesn't feel that their thyroid management is optimal, consider giving your medical provider a copy of the commentary.

If he or she is unwilling to entertain these recommendations or guidelines, then unfortunately, it may be time for you to look for another provider who will.

We can do better! It is time.

BIBLIOGRAPHY

INTRODUCTION

1. Vanderpump, M. P., Tunbridge, W. M., French, J. M., Appleton, D., Bates, D., Clark, F., Grimley Evans, J., Hasan, D. M., Rodgers, H., Tunbridge, F., et al. "The Incidence of Thyroid Disorders in the Community: A Twenty-year Follow-Up of the Whickham Survey." *Clinical Endocrinology (Oxford)* 43, no. 1 (1995): 55-68. doi: 10.1111/j.1365-2265.1995.tb01894.x. PMID: 7641412.

2. Hollowell, J. G., Staehling, N. W., Flanders, W. D., Hannon, W. H., Gunter, E. W., Spencer, C. A., Braverman, L. E. "Serum TSH, T(4), and Thyroid Antibodies in the United States Population (1988 to 1994): National Health and Nutrition Examination Survey (NHANES III)." *The Journal of Clinical Endocrinology & Metabolism* 87, no. 2 (2002): 489-99. doi: 10.1210/jcem.87.2.8182. PMID: 11836274.

3. Sawin, C. T., Castelli, W. P., Hershman, J. M., McNamara, P., Bacharach, P. "The Aging Thyroid. Thyroid Deficiency in the Framingham Study." *Archives of Internal Medicine* 145, no. 8 (1985): 1386-1388. PMID: 4026469.

CHAPTER 1

1. Jonklaas, J., Bianco, A. C., Bauer, A. J., Burman, K. D., Cappola, A. R., Celi, F. S., Cooper, D. S., Kim B. W., Peeters, R. P., Rosenthal, M. S., Sawka, A. M.; American Thyroid Association Task Force on Thyroid Hormone Replacement. "Guidelines for the Treatment of Hypothyroidism: Prepared by the American Thyroid Association Task Force on Thyroid Hormone Replacement." *Thyroid* 24, no. 12 (2014): 1670-1751. doi: 10.1089/thy.2014.0028. PMID: 25266247; PMCID: PMC4267409.

2. Kalra, S., Khandelwal, S. K. "Why Are Our Hypothyroid Patients Unhappy? Is Tissue Hypothyroidism the Answer?" *Indian Journal of Endocrinology and Metabolism* 15, no. 2 Suppl (2011): S95-98. doi: 10.4103/2230-8210.83333. PMID: 21966661; PMCID: PMC3169863.

3. "Goiter." American Thyroid Association. URL: https://www.thyroid.org/goiter/.

4. Salisbury, S. "Cretinism: The Past, Present and Future of Diagnosis and Cure." *Paediatrics & Child Health* 8, no. 2 (2003): 105-106. doi: 10.1093/pch/8.2.105. PMID: 20019927; PMCID: PMC2791432.

5. "Myxedema." ScienceDirect. URL: https://www.sciencedirect.com/topics/pharmacology-toxicology-and-pharmaceutical-science/myxedema/.

6. Hanney, S. R., Castle-Clarke, S., Grant, J. et al. "How Long Does Biomedical Research Take? Studying the Time Taken Between Biomedical and Health Research and its Translation into Products, Policy, and Practice." *Health Research Policy and Systems* 13, no. 1 (2015). URL: https://doi.org/10.1186/1478-4505-13-1/.

7. Smith, S. R. "Desiccated Thyroid Preparations: Obsolete Therapy." *Archives of Internal Medicine* 144, no. 5 (1984): 926–927. doi:10.1001/archinte.1984.00350170062009.

8. Ortiga-Carvalho, T. M., Sidhaye, A. R., Wondisford, F. E. "Thyroid Hormone Receptors and Resistance to Thyroid Hormone Disorders." *Nature Reviews Endocrinology* 10, no. 10 (2014): 582-591. doi: 10.1038/nrendo.2014.143. Epub 2014 Aug 19. PMID: 25135573; PMCID: PMC4578869.

9. Midgley, J. E., Larisch, R., Dietrich, J. W., Hoermann, R. "Variation in the Biochemical Response toL-Thyroxine Therapy and Relationship with Peripheral Thyroid Hormone Conversion Efficiency." *Endocrine Connections* 4, no 4 (2015): 196-205. doi: 10.1530/ec-150056. PMID: 26335522; PMCID: PMC4557078.

CHAPTER 2

1. Schectman, J. M., Kallenberg, G. A., Hirsch, R. P., Shumacher, R. J. "Report of an Association Between Race and Thyroid Stimulating Hormone Level." *American Journal of Public Health* 81, no. 4 (1991): 505-506. doi: 10.2105/ajph.81.4.505. PMID: 2003636; PMCID: PMC1405055.

2. Oh, J. Y., Sung, Y. A., Lee, H. J. "Elevated Thyroid Stimulating Hormone Levels are Associated with Metabolic Syndrome in Euthyroid Young Women." *Korean Journal of Internal Medicine* 228, no. 2 (2013): 180-186. doi: 10.3904/kjim.2013.28.2.180. Epub 2013 Feb 27. PMID: 23525791; PMCID: PMC3604608.

3. Sheehan, M. T. "Biochemical Testing of the Thyroid: TSH is the Best and, Oftentimes, Only Test Needed - A Review for Primary Care." *Clinical Medicine Research* 14, no. 2 (2016): 83-92. doi: 10.3121/cmr.2016.1309. Epub 2016 May 26. PMID: 27231117; PMCID: PMC5321289.

4. Alevizaki, M., Mantzou, E., Cimponeriu, A. T., Alevizaki, C. C., Koutras, D. A. "TSH May Not Be a Good Marker for Adequate Thyroid Hormone Replacement Therapy." *Wiener Klinische Wochenschrift* 117, no. 18 (2005): 636-640. doi: 10.1007/s00508-005-0421-0. PMID: 16416346.

5. Liu, G., Liang, L., Bray, G. A., Qi, L., Hu, F. B., Rood, J., Sacks, F. M., Sun, Q. "Thyroid Hormones and Changes in Body Weight and Metabolic Parameters in Response to Weight Loss Diets: The POUNDS LOST Trial." *International Journal of Obesity (London)* 41, no. 6 (2017): 878-886. doi: 10.1038/ijo.2017.28. Epub 2017 Jan 31. PMID: 28138133; PMCID: PMC5461198.

6. Tibaldi, J. M., Surks, M. I. "Effects of Nonthyroidal Illness on Thyroid Function." *Medical Clinics of North America* 69, no. 5 (1985): 899-911. doi: 10.1016/s0025-7125(16)30996-8. PMID: 3932793.

7. Tibaldi, J. M., Surks, M. I. "Effects of Nonthyroidal Illness on Thyroid Function." *Medical Clinic of North America* 69, no. 5 (1985): 899-911. doi: 10.1016/s0025-7125(16)30996-8. PMID: 3932793.

8. DeGroot, L. J. "The Non-Thyroidal Illness Syndrome." Updated 2015 Feb 1. In *Endotext* [Internet]. South Dartmouth (MA): MDText.com, Inc.; 2000-. Available from: https://www.ncbi.nlm.nih.gov/books/NBK285570/.

9. Mehran, L., Tohidi, M., Sarvghadi, F., Delshad, H., Amouzegar, A., Soldin, O. P., Azizi, F. "Management of Thyroid Peroxidase Antibody Euthyroid Women in Pregnancy: Comparison of the American Thyroid Association and the Endocrine Society Guidelines." *Journal of Thyroid Research*. 2013 (2013): 542692. doi: 10.1155/2013/542692. Epub 2013 May 12. PMID: 23738229; PMCID: PMC3666229.

10. Fröhlich, E., Wahl, R. "Thyroid Autoimmunity: Role of Antithyroid Antibodies in Thyroid and Extra-Thyroidal Diseases." *Frontiers in Immunology* 8 (2017): 521. doi: 10.3389/fimmu.2017.00521. PMID: 28536577; PMCID: PMC5422478.

11. Staub, J. J., Conti, A., Huber, P., Martens, M., Ackermann, F., Müller-Brand, J., Kofler, C. "Sexhormonbindendes Globulin (SHBG), Ein Neuer Metabolischer In-vitro-Test der Schilddrüsenfunktion [Sex Hormone Binding Globulin (SHBG), a New Metabolic in Vitro Thyroid Function Test]." *Schweizerische Medizinische Wochenschrift* 108, no. 48 (1978): 1909-1911. German. PMID: 568820.

CHAPTER 3

1. Dunta, B. "A Renewed Focus on The Association Between Thyroid Hormones and Lipid Metabolism." *Frontiers in Endocrinology* 9 (2018): 1664-2392.

2. Sathi, P., Kalyan, S., Hitchcock, C.L., Pudek, M., Prior J. C. "Progesterone Therapy Increases Free Thyroxine Levels--Data from a Randomized Placebo-Controlled 12-Week Hot Fush Trial." *Clinical Endocrinology (Oxford)* 79, no. 2 (2013): 282-287. doi: 10.1111/cen.12128. Epub 2013 May 6. PMID: 23252963.

3. Koehler, V. F., Mann, U., Nassour, A., Mann, W. A. "Fake News? Biotin Interference in Thyroid Immunoassays." *Clinical Chimica Acta* 484 (2018): 320-322. doi: 10.1016/j.cca.2018.05.053. Epub 2018 May 30. PMID: 29856977.

CHAPTER 4

1. Ganesan, K., Wadud, K. "Euthyroid, Sick Syndrome." Updated 2021 Oct 30. In: *StatPearls* [Internet]. Treasure Island (FL): StatPearls Publishing; 2022 Jan-. Available from: https://www.ncbi.nlm.nih.gov/books/NBK482219/.

CHAPTER 5

1. Hollowell, J. G., Staehling, N. W., Flanders, W. D., Hannon, W. H., Gunter, E. W., Spencer, C. A., Braverman, L. E. "Serum TSH, T(4), and Thyroid Antibodies in the United States Population (1988 to 1994): National Health and Nutrition

Examination Survey (NHANES III)." *The Journal of Clinical Endocrinology & Metabolism* 87, no. 2 (2002): 489-499. doi: 10.1210/jcem.87.2.8182. PMID: 11836274.

2. Martinez, O. M., Krams, S. M. "The Immune Response to Epstein Barr Virus and Implications for Posttransplant Lymphoproliferative Disorder." *Transplantation.* 101, no. 9 (2017): 2009-2016. doi: 10.1097/TP.0000000000001767. PMID: 28376031; PMCID: PMC5568952.

3. Ni, H. K., Liao, L. M., Huang, R. L., Zhou, W. "The Relationship Between Gastric Cancer and Helicobacter Pylori Cytotoxin-Related Gene A Genotypes." *Cellular and Molecular Biology (Noisy-le-grand)* 66, no. 7 (2020): 1-4. PMID: 33287914.

4. "Helicobacter pylori (H. pylori) infection." Mayo Clinic. URL: https://www.mayoclinic.org/diseases-conditions/h-pylori/diagnosis-treatment/drc-20356177

5. Murdaca, G., Tonacci, A., Negrini, S., Greco, M., Borro, M., Puppo, F., Gangemi, S. "Emerging Role of Vitamin D in Autoimmune Diseases: An Update on Evidence and Therapeutic Implications." *Autoimmunity Reviews* 18, no. 9 (2019): 102350. doi: 10.1016/j.autrev.2019.102350. Epub 2019 Jul 16. PMID: 31323357.

6. Sanna, A., Firinu, D., Zavattari, P., Valera, P. "Zinc Status and Autoimmunity: A Systematic Review and Meta-Analysis." *Nutrients* 10, no. 1 (2018): 68. doi: 10.3390/nu10010068. PMID: 29324654; PMCID: PMC5793296.

7. Gärtner, R., Gasnier, B. C., Dietrich, J. W., Krebs, B., Angstwurm, M. W. "Selenium Supplementation in Patients with Autoimmune Thyroiditis Decreases Thyroid Peroxidase Antibodies Concentrations." *The Journal of Clinical Endocrinology & Metabolism* 87, no. 4 (2002): 1687-1691. doi: 10.1210/jcem.87.4.8421. PMID: 11932302.

8. Arteel, G. E., Sies, H. "The Biochemistry of Selenium and the Glutathione System." *Environmental Toxicology and Pharmacology*. 10, no. 4 (2001): 153-158. doi: 10.1016/s1382-6689(01)00078-3. PMID: 21782571.

9. "The Microbiome." Harvard T.H. Chan School of Public Health. URL: https://www.hsph.harvard.edu/nutritionsource/microbiome/.

10. Liu, S., An, Y., Cao, B., Sun, R., Ke, J., Zhao, D. "The Composition of Gut Microbiota in Patients Bearing Hashimoto's Thyroiditis with Euthyroidism and Hypothyroidism." *International Journal of Endocrinology* 10 (2020): 5036959. doi: 10.1155/2020/5036959. PMID: 33224194; PMCID: PMC7673947.

11. Patil, A. D. "Link Between Hypothyroidism and Small Intestinal Bacterial Overgrowth." *Indian Journal of Endocrinology and Metabolism* 18, no. 3 (2014): 307-309. doi: 10.4103/2230-8210.131155. PMID: 24944923; PMCID: PMC4056127.

12. Rojas, M., Restrepo-Jiménez, P., Monsalve, D. M., Pacheco, Y., Acosta-Ampudia, Y., Ramírez-Santana, C., Leung, P. S. C., Ansari, A. A., Gershwin, M. E., Anaya, J. M. "Molecular Mimicry and Autoimmunity." *Journal of Autoimmunity* 95 (2018): 100-123. doi: 10.1016/j.jaut.2018.10.012. Epub 2018 Oct 26. PMID: 30509385.

13. Catassi, C., Elli, L., Bonaz, B., Bouma, G., Carroccio, A., Castillejo, G., Cellier, C., Cristofori, F., de Magistris, L., Dolinsek, J., Dieterich, W., Francavilla, R., Hadjivassiliou, M., Holtmeier, W., Körner, U., Leffler, D. A., Lundin, K. E., Mazzarella, G., Mulder, C. J., Pellegrini, N., Rostami, K., Sanders, D., Skodje, G. I., Schuppan D., Ullrich R., Volta U., Williams M., Zevallos V. F., Zopf Y., Fasano A. "Diagnosis of Non-Celiac Gluten Sensitivity (NCGS): The Salerno Experts' Criteria." *Nutrients* 7, no. 6 (2015): 4966-4977. doi: 10.3390/nu7064966. PMID: 26096570; PMCID: PMC4488826.

14. Zaletel, K., Gaberšček, S. "Hashimoto's Thyroiditis: From Genes to the Disease." *Current Genomics* 12, no. 8 (2011): 576-588. doi: 10.2174/138920211798120763. PMID: 22654557; PMCID: PMC3271310.

15. Straub, R. H. "Interaction of the Endocrine System with Inflammation: A Function of Energy and Volume Regulation." *Arthritis Research & Therapy* 16, no. 1 (2014): 203. doi: 10.1186/ar4484. PMID: 24524669; PMCID: PMC3978663.

16. Shoelson, S. E, Lee, J., Goldfine, A. B. "Inflammation and Insulin Resistance." *Journal of Clinical Investigation* 116, no. 7 (2006): 1793-801. doi: 10.1172/JCI29069. Erratum in: *Journal of Clinical Investigation* 116, no. 8 (2006): 2308. PMID: 16823477; PMCID: PMC1483173.

17. Ch'ng, C. L., Jones, M. K., Kingham, J. G. "Celiac Disease and Autoimmune Thyroid Disease." *Clinical Medicine & Research* 5, no. 3 (2007): 184-192. doi: 10.3121/cmr.2007.738. PMID: 18056028; PMCID: PMC2111403.

18. Carta, M. G., Loviselli, A., Hardoy, M. C., Massa, S., Cadeddu, M., Sardu, C., Carpiniello, B., Dell'Osso, L., Mariotti, S. "The Link Between Thyroid Autoimmunity (Antithyroid Peroxidase Autoantibodies) with Anxiety and Mood Disorders in the Community: A Feld of Interest for Public Health in the Future." *BMC Psychiatry* 4 (2004): 25. doi: 10.1186/1471-244X-4-25. PMID: 15317653; PMCID: PMC516779.

19. "Hashimoto Thyroiditis Treatment & Management." eMedicine. URL: https://emedicine.medscape.com/article/120937-treatment

20. Fröhlich, E., Wahl, R. "Thyroid Autoimmunity: Role of Anti-thyroid Antibodies in Thyroid and Extra-Thyroidal Diseases." *Frontiers in Immunology* 8 (2017): 521. doi: 10.3389/fimmu.2017.00521. PMID: 28536577; PMCID: PMC5422478.

21. Konijeti, G. G., Kim, N., Lewis, J. D., Groven, S., Chandrasekaran, A., Grandhe, S., Diamant, C., Singh, E., Oliveira, G., Wang, X., Molparia, B., Torkamani, A. "Efficacy of the Autoimmune Protocol Diet for Inflammatory Bowel Disease." *Inflammatory Bowel Diseases* 23, no. 11 (2017): 2054-2060. doi: 10.1097/MIB.0000000000001221. PMID: 28858071; PMCID: PMC5647120.

22. Asik, M., Gunes, F., Binnetoglu, E., Eroglu, M., Bozkurt, N., Sen, H., Akbal, E., Bakar, C., Beyazit, Y., Ukinc, K. "Decrease in TSH Levels After Lactose Restriction in Hashimoto's Thyroiditis Patients with Lactose Intolerance." *Endocrine* 46, no. 2 (2014): 279-284. doi: 10.1007/s12020-013-0065-1. PMID: 24078411.

23. Prasad, A. S. "Zinc is an Antioxidant and Anti-Inflammatory Agent: Its Role in Human Health." *Frontiers in Nutrition* 1 (2014): 14. doi: 10.3389/fnut.2014.00014. PMID: 25988117; PMCID: PMC4429650.

24. Shankar, A. H., Prasad, A. S. "Zinc and Immune Function: The Biological Basis of Altered Resistance to Infection." *American Journal of Clinical Nutrition* 68, no. 2 Suppl (1998): 447S-463S. doi: 10.1093/ajcn/68.2.447S. PMID: 9701160.

25. Olivieri, O., Girelli, D., Stanzial, A. M., Rossi, L., Bassi, A., Corrocher, R. "Selenium, Zinc, and Thyroid Hormones in Healthy Subjects: Low T3/T4 Ratio in the Elderly is Related to Impaired Selenium Status." *Biological Trace Element Research* 51, no. 1 (1996): 31-41. doi: 10.1007/BF02790145. PMID: 8834378.

26. Drutel, A., Archambeaud, F., Caron, P. "Selenium and the Thyroid Gland: More Good News for Clinicians." *Clinical Endocrinology (Oxford)* 78, no. 2 (2013): 155-164. doi: 10.1111/cen.12066. PMID: 23046013.

27. Walter, K. N., Corwin, E. J., Ulbrecht, J., Demers, L. M., Bennett, J. M., Whetzel, C. A., Klein, L. C. "Elevated Thyroid Stimulating Hormone is Associated with Elevated Cortisol in Healthy Young Men and Women." *Thyroid Research* 5, no. 1 (2012): 13. doi: 10.1186/1756-6614-5-13. PMID: 23111240; PMCID: PMC3520819.

28. Talaei, A., Ghorbani, F., Asemi, Z. "The Effects of Vitamin D Supplementation on Thyroid Function in Hypothyroid Patients: A Randomized, Double-blind, Placebo-Controlled Trial." *Indian Journal of Endocrinology and Metabolism* 22, no. 5 (2018): 584-588. doi: 10.4103/ijem.IJEM_603_17. PMID: 30294564; PMCID: PMC6166548.

29. Kim, D. "The Role of Vitamin D in Thyroid Diseases." *Internatonal Journal of Molecular Sciences* 18, no. 9 (2017): 1949. doi: 10.3390/ijms18091949. PMID: 28895880; PMCID: PMC5618598.

30. Younger, J., Parkitny, L., McLain, D. "The Use of Low-Dose Naltrexone (LDN) as a Novel Anti-Inflammatory Treatment for Chronic Pain." *Clinical Rheumatology* 33, no. 4 (2014): 451-459. doi: 10.1007/s10067-014-2517-2. Epub 2014 Feb 15. PMID: 24526250; PMCID: PMC3962576.

31. Ilias, I., Kakoulas, I., Christakopoulou, I., Katsadoros, K. "Thyroid Function of Former Opioid Addicts on Naltrexone Treatment." *Acta Medica* (Hradec Kralove) 44, no. 1 (2001): 33-35. PMID: 11367890.

32. Bihari, B., "Bernard Bihari, MD: Low-Dose Naltrexone for Normalizing Immune System Function." *Alternative Therapies in Health and Medicine* 19, no. 2 (2013): 56-65. PMID: 23594453.

33. Black, D. S., Slavich, G. M. "Mindfulness Meditation and the Immune System: A Systematic Review of Randomized Controlled Trials." *Annals of the New York Academy Sciences* 1373, no. 1 (2016): 13-24. doi: 10.1111/nyas.12998. Epub 2016 Jan 21. PMID: 26799456; PMCID: PMC4940234.

34. Campbell, A. W. "Autoimmunity and the Gut." *Autoimmune Diseases* (2014): 152428. doi: 10.1155/2014/152428. Epub 2014 May 13. PMID: 24900918; PMCID: PMC4036413.

35. Krysiak, R., Kowalcze, K., Okopień, B. "The effect of testosterone on thyroid autoimmunity in euthyroid men with Hashimoto's thyroiditis and low testosterone levels." *Journal of Clinical Pharmacy and Therapeutics* 44, no. 5 (2019): 742-749. doi: 10.1111/jcpt.12987. Epub 2019 Jun 10. PMID: 31183891.

36. Takasu, N., Komiya, I., Asawa, T., Nagasawa, Y., Yamada, T. "Test for Recovery from Hypothyroidism During Thyroxine Therapy in Hashimoto's Thyroiditis." *The Lancet* 336, no. 8723 (1990): 1084-1086. doi: 10.1016/0140-6736(90)92567-2. PMID: 1977978.

37. National Library of Medicine. URL: https://www.ncbi.nlm.nih. gov/pmc/articles/PMC5112739/.

38. National Library of Medicine. URL: https://www.ncbi.nlm.nih. gov/pmc/articles/PMC5870944/.

CHAPTER 6

1. Naji Rad, S., Deluxe, L. "Postpartum Thyroiditis." Updated 2022 Jun 21. In: *StatPearls* [Internet]. Treasure Island (FL): StatPearls Publishing; 2022 Jan-. Available from: https://www. ncbi.nlm.nih.gov/books/NBK557646/.

2. Arnason, T., Clarke, D. B., Imran, S. A. "Hyperthyroidism Caused by a Pituitary Adenoma." *CMAJ* 183, no. 11 (2011): E757. doi: 10.1503/cmaj.101244. Epub 2011 Apr 4. PMID: 21464161; PMCID: PMC3153549.

3. Fu, J., Wu, A., Wang, X., Guan, H. "Concurrent Graves' Disease and TSH Secreting Pituitary Adenoma Presenting Suppressed Thyrotropin Levels: A Case Report and Review of the Literature." *Frontiers in Endocrinology (Lausanne)* 11 (2020): 523. doi: 10.3389/fendo.2020.00523. PMID: 32849306; PMCID: PMC7424009.

4. Medas, F., Erdas, E., Canu, G. L. *et al.* "Does Hyperthyroidism Worsen the Prognosis of Thyroid Carcinoma? A Retrospective Analysis on 2820 Consecutive Thyroidectomies." *Journal of Otolaryngology - Head & Neck Surgery* 47, no. 6 (2018). URL: https://doi.org/10.1186/s40463-018-0254-2/.

5. DeGroot, L. J. "Diagnosis and Treatment of Graves' Disease." Updated 2016 Nov 2. In: Feingold KR, Anawalt B, Boyce A, et al., editors. *Endotext* [Internet]. South Dartmouth (MA): MDText.com, Inc.; 2000-. Available from: https://www.ncbi.nlm.nih.gov/books/NBK285548/.

6. Pyzik, A., Grywalska, E., Matyjaszek-Matuszek, B., Ludian, J., Kiszczak-Bochyńska, E., Smoleń, A., Roliński, J., Pyzik, D. "Does the Epstein-Barr Virus Play a Role in the Pathogenesis of Graves' Disease?" *International Journal of Molecular Sciences* 20, no. 13 (2019): 3145. doi: 10.3390/ijms20133145. PMID: 31252621; PMCID: PMC6650880.

7. LiVolsi, V. A., Baloch, Z. W. "The Pathology of Hyperthyroidism." *Frontiers in Endocrinology (Lausanne)* 9 (2018): 737. doi: 10.3389/fendo.2018.00737. PMID: 30559722; PMCID: PMC6286962.

8. Leung, A. M., Braverman L. E. "Consequences of Excess Iodine." *Nature Reviews Endocrinology* 10, no. 3 (2014): 136-142. doi: 10.1038/nrendo.2013.251. Epub 2013 Dec 17. PMID: 24342882; PMCID: PMC3976240.

9. Mullur, R., Liu, Y. Y., Brent, G. A. "Thyroid Hormone Regulation of Metabolism." *Physiological Reviews* 94, no. 2 (2014): 355-382. doi: 10.1152/physrev.00030.2013. PMID: 24692351; PMCID: PMC4044302.

10. Bielecka-Dabrowa, A., Mikhailidis, D. P., Rysz, J., Banach, M. "The Mechanisms of Atrial Fbrillation in Hyperthyroidism." *Thyroid Research* 2, no. 1 (2009): 4. doi: 10.1186/1756-6614-2-4. PMID: 19341475; PMCID: PMC2680813.

11. Saito, J., Nishikawa, T. "[Osteoporosis Treatment in Patients with Hyperthyroidism]." *Nihon Rinsho* 67, no. 5 (2009): 1011-1016. Japanese. PMID: 19432125.

12. McKenzie, J. M., Zakarija, M. "A Reconsideration of a Thyroid-Stimulating Immunoglobulin as the Cause of Hyperthyroidism in Graves' Disease." *The Journal of Clinical Endocrinology & Metabolism* 42, no. 4 (1976): 778-781. doi: 10.1210/jcem-42-4-778. PMID: 177449.

13. Luttrell, B. M., Hales, I. B. "Thyroid Stimulating Immunoglobulin in Graves' Disease." *Australian and New Zealand Journal of Medicine* 11, no. 3 (1981): 293-298. PMID: 6170289.

14. Pokhrel, B., Aiman, W., Bhusal, K. "Thyroid Storm." Updated 2022 Oct 6. In: *StatPearls* [Internet]. Treasure Island (FL): StatPearls Publishing; 2022 Jan-. Available from: https://www.ncbi.nlm.nih.gov/books/NBK448095/.

15. Wiersinga, W. M. "Propranolol and Thyroid Hormone Metabolism." *Thyroid* 1, no. 3 (1991): 273-277. doi: 10.1089/thy.1991.1.273. PMID: 1688102.

16. Abraham, P., Acharya, S. "Current and Emerging Treatment Options for Graves' Hyperthyroidism." *Therapeutics and Clinical Risk Management* 6 (2010): 29-40. doi: 10.2147/tcrm.s5229. PMID: 20169034; PMCID: PMC2817786.

17. Azizi, F., Yousefi, V., Bahrainian, A., Sheikholeslami, F., Tohidi, M., Mehrabi, Y. "Long-Term Continuous Methimazole or Radioiodine Treatment for Hyperthyroidism." *Archives of Iranian Medicine* 15, no. 8 (2012): 477-484. PMID: 22827783.

18. Tatara, M. R., Gołyński, M., Radzki, R. P., Bieńko, M., Krupski, W. "Effects of Long-Term Oral Administration of Methimazole on Femur and Tibia Properties in Male Wistar Rats." *Biomedicine & Pharmacotherapy* 94 (2017): 124-128. doi: 10.1016/j.biopha.2017.07.107. Epub 2017 Jul 28. PMID: 28759749.

19. Moretto, R. L., Pedro, A. B., Leite, A. C., Romaldini, J. H. "Avaliação do Peso Corporal em Pacientes com Doença de Graves Durante o Tratamento com Metimazol [Evaluation of Body Weight in Patients with Graves' Disease During the Treatment with Methimazole]." *Arquivos Brasileiros de Endocrinologia & Metabologia* 56, no. 6 (2012): 364-369. Portuguese. doi: 10.1590/s0004-27302012000600004. PMID: 22990640.

20. Szumowski, P., Mojsak, M., Abdelrazek, S., Sykała, M., Amelian-Fiłonowicz, A., Jurgilewicz, D., Myśliwiec, J. "Calculation of Therapeutic Activity of Radioiodine in Graves' Disease by Means of Marinelli's Formula, Using Technetium (^{99m}Tc) Scintigraphy." *Endocrine* 54, no. 3 (2016): 751-756. doi: 10.1007/s12020-016-1074-7. Epub 2016 Aug 24. PMID: 27553050; PMCID: PMC5566489.

21. Wiersinga, W. M. "Graves' Disease: Can It Be Cured?" *Endocrinology and Metabolism (Seoul)* 34, no. 1 (2019): 29-38. doi: 10.3803/EnM.2019.34.1.29. PMID: 30912336; PMCID: PMC6435849.

22. Zen, X. X., Yuan, Y., Liu, Y., Wu, T. X., Han, S. "Chinese Herbal Medicines for Hyperthyroidism." *Cochrane Database of Systematic Reviews* 2007, no. 2 (2007): CD005450. doi: 10.1002/14651858.CD005450.pub2. PMID: 17443591; PMCID: PMC6544778.

23. Ch'ng, C. L., Jones, M. K., Kingham, J. G. "Celiac Disease and Autoimmune Thyroid Disease." *Clinical Medicine & Research* 5, no. 3 (2007): 184-192. doi: 10.3121/cmr.2007.738. PMID: 18056028; PMCID: PMC2111403.

24. Prasad, A. S. "Zinc in Human Health: Effect of Zinc on Immune Cells." *Molecular Medicine* 14, no. 5-6 (2008): 353-357. doi: 10.2119/2008-00033.Prasad. PMID: 18385818; PMCID: PMC2277319.

25. Prasad, A. S. "Zinc is an Antioxidant and Anti-Inflammatory Agent: Its Role in Human Health." *Frontiers in Nutrition* 1 (2014): 14. doi: 10.3389/fnut.2014.00014. PMID: 25988117; PMCID: PMC4429650.

26. Betsy, A., Binitha, M., Sarita, S. "Zinc Deficiency Associated with Hypothyroidism: An Overlooked Cause of Severe Alopecia." *International Journal of Trichology* 5, no. 1 (2013): 40-42. doi: 10.4103/0974-7753.114714. PMID: 23960398; PMCID: PMC3746228.

27. Alhuzaim, O. N., Aljohani, N. "Effect of Vitamin D3 on Untreated Graves' Disease with Vitamin D Deficiency." *Clinical Medicine Insights: Case Reports* 7 (2014): 83-85. doi: 10.4137/CCRep.S13157. PMID: 25187748; PMCID: PMC4133032.

28. Maroon, J. C., Bost, J. W. "Omega-3 Fatty Acids (Fish Oil) as an Anti-Inflammatory: An Alternative to Nonsteroidal Anti-Inflammatory Drugs for Discogenic Pain." *Surgical Neurology* 65, no. 4 (2006): 326-331. doi: 10.1016/j.surneu.2005.10.023. PMID: 16531187.

29. Jones, J. E., Desper, P. C., Shane, S. R., Flink, E. B. "Magnesium Metabolism in Hyperthyroidism and Hypothyroidism." *Journal of Clinical Investigation* 45, no. 6 (1966): 891-900. doi: 10.1172/JCI105404. PMID: 5913297; PMCID: PMC292768.

30. Galland, L. "Magnesium and Immune Function: An Overview." *Magnesium* 7, no. 5-6 (1988): 290-299. PMID: 3075245.

31. Leung, A. M., Braverman, L. E. "Consequences of Excess Iodine." *Nature Reviews Endocrinology* 10, no. 3 (2014): 136-142. doi: 10.1038/nrendo.2013.251. Epub 2013 Dec 17. PMID: 24342882; PMCID: PMC3976240.

32. Panossian, A., Wikman, G. "Effects of Adaptogens on the Central Nervous System and the Molecular Mechanisms Associated with Their Stress-Protective Activity." *Pharmaceuticals* (Basel) 3, no. 1 (2010): 188-224. doi: 10.3390/ph3010188. PMID: 27713248; PMCID: PMC3991026.

33. Kaplan, D., Dosiou, C. "Two Cases of Graves' Hyperthyroidism Treated with Homeopathic Remedies Containing Herbal Extracts from *Lycopus spp.* And *Melissa officinalis.*" *Journal of the Endocrine Society* 5, no. 1 Suppl (2021): A971. doi: 10.1210/jendso/bvab048.1984. PMCID: PMC8090196.

34. Anton, R. F. "Naltrexone for the Management of Alcohol Dependence." *New England Journal of Medicine* 359, no. 7 (2008): 715-721. doi: 10.1056/NEJMct0801733. PMID: 18703474; PMCID: PMC2565602.

35. Segal, D., Macdonald, J. K., Chande, N. "Low Dose Naltrexone for Induction of Remission in Crohn's Disease." *Cochrane Database of Systematic Reviews* 2 (2014): CD010410. doi:

10.1002/14651858.CD010410.pub2. Update in: Cochrane Database Syst Rev. 2018 Apr 01;4:CD010410. PMID: 24558033.

36. Li, J., Bai, L., Wei, F., et al. "Effect of Addition of Thyroxine in the Treatment of Graves' Disease: A Systematic Review." *Frontiers in Endocrinology*. 25 January 2021. Section Thyroid Endocrinology.

37. Wiersinga W. M. "Graves' Disease: Can It Be Cured?" *Endocrinology and Metababolism (Seoul)* 34, no. 1 (2019): 29-38. doi: 10.3803/ EnM.2019.34.1.29. PMID: 30912336; PMCID: PMC6435849.

38. Butt S., Patel B. C. "Exophthalmos." Updated 2022 Jun 27. In: *StatPearls* [Internet]. Treasure Island (FL): StatPearls Publishing; 2022 Jan-. Available from: https://www.ncbi.nlm.nih.gov/ books/NBK559323/.

CHAPTER 7

1. Gullo, D., Latina, A., Frasca, F., Le Moli, R., Pellegriti, G., Vigneri, R. "Levothyroxine Monotherapy Cannot Guarantee Euthyroidism in All Athyreotic Patients." *PLOS ONE* 6, no. 8 (2011): e22552. doi: 10.1371/journal.pone.0022552. Epub 2011 Aug 1. PMID: 21829633; PMCID: PMC3148220.

2. Jonklaas, J., Nsouli-Maktabi, H. "Weight Changes in Euthyroid Patients Undergoing Thyroidectomy." *Thyroid* 21, no. 12 (2011): 1343-1351. doi: 10.1089/thy.2011.0054. Epub 2011 Nov 8. PMID: 22066482; PMCID: PMC3229816.

CHAPTER 8

1. Dean, D. S., Gharib, H. "Epidemiology of Thyroid Nodules." *Best Practice and Research Clinical Endocrinology & Metabolism* 22, no. 6 (2008): 901-911. doi: 10.1016/j.beem.2008.09.019. PMID: 19041821.

2. Bomeli, S. R., LeBeau, S. O., Ferris, R. L. "Evaluation of a Thyroid Nodule." *Otolaryngologic Clinics of North America* 43, no. 2 (2010): 229-238, vii. doi: 10.1016/j.otc.2010.01.002. PMID: 20510711; PMCID: PMC2879398.

3. Popoveniuc, G., Jonklaas, J. "Thyroid Nodules." *Medical Clinics of North America* 96, no. 2 (2012): 329-349. doi: 10.1016/j. mcna.2012.02.002. PMID: 22443979; PMCID: PMC3575959.

4. Resende de Paiva, C, Grønhøj, C, Feldt-Rasmussen, U, von Buchwald, C. "Association between Hashimoto's Thyroiditis and Thyroid Cancer in 64,628 Patients." *Frontiers in Oncology* 7 (2017): 53. doi: 10.3389/fonc.2017.00053. PMID: 28443243; PMCID: PMC5385456.

5. Nikiforov, Y. E. "Is Ionizing Radiation Responsible for the Increasing Incidence of Thyroid Cancer?" *Cancer* 116, no. 7 (2010): 1626-1628. doi: 10.1002/cncr.24889. PMID: 20151420; PMCID: PMC2847020.

6. Brito, J. P., Gionfriddo, M. R., Al Nofal, A., Boehmer, K. R., Leppin, A. L., Reading, C., Callstrom, M., Elraiyah, T. A., Prokop, L. J., Stan, M. N., Murad, M. H., Morris, J. C., Montori, V. M. "The Accuracy of Thyroid Nodule Ultrasound to Predict Thyroid Cancer: Systematic Review and Meta-analysis." *The Journal of Clinical Endocrinology & Metabolism* 99, no. 4 (2014): 1253-1263. doi: 10.1210/jc.2013-2928. Epub 2013 Nov 25. PMID: 24276450; PMCID: PMC3973781.

7. Golbert, L., de Cristo, A. P., Faccin, C. S., Farenzena, M., Folgierini, H., Graudenz, M. S., Maia, A. L. "Serum TSH Levels as a Predictor of Malignancy in Thyroid Nodules: A Prospective Study." *PLOS ONE* 12, no. 11 (2017): e0188123. doi: 10.1371/journal.pone.0188123. PMID: 29145466; PMCID: PMC5690674.

8. Hannoush, Z. C., Weiss, R. E. "Thyroid Hormone Replacement in Patients Following Thyroidectomy for Thyroid Cancer." *Rambam Maimonides Medical Journal* 7, no. 1 (2016): e0002. doi: 10.5041/RMMJ.10229. PMID: 26886951; PMCID: PMC4737508.

9. Rivas, A. M., Lado-Abeal, J. "Thyroid Hormone Resistance and its Management." *Proceedings (Baylor University Medical Center)* 29, no. 2 (2016): 209-211. doi: 10.1080/08998280.2016.11929421. PMID: 27034574; PMCID: PMC4790576.

CHAPTER 9

1. Sapin, R., Schlienger, J. L. "Dosages de Thyroxine (T4) et Tri-Iodothyronine (T3): Techniques et Place dans le Bilan Thyroïdien Fonctionnel [Thyroxine (T4) and Tri-Iodothyronine (T3) Determinations: Techniques and Value in the Assessment of Thyroid Function]." *Annales de Biologie Clinique (Paris)* 61, no. 4 (2003): 411-420. French. PMID: 12915350.

2. Vijay Panicker, Ponnusamy Saravanan, Bijay Vaidya, Jonathan Evans, Andrew T. Hattersley, Timothy M. Frayling, Colin M. Dayan, "Common Variation in the *DIO2* Gene Predicts Baseline Psychological Well-Being and Response to Combination Thyroxine Plus Triiodothyronine Therapy in Hypothyroid Patients." *The Journal of Clinical Endocrinology & Metabolism* 94,no. 5 (2009): 1623–1629. URL: https://doi.org/10.1210/jc.2008-1301/.

3. Kalász, H., Antal, I. "Drug Excipients." *Current Medicinal Chemistry* 13, no. 21 (2006): 2535-2563. doi: 10.2174/092986706778201648. PMID: 17017910.

4. Muñoz-Torres, M., Varsavsky, M., Alonso, G. "Lactose Intolerance Revealed by Severe Resistance to Treatment with Levothyroxine." *Thyroid* 16, no. 11 (2006): 1171-1173. doi: 10.1089/thy.2006.16.1171. PMID: 17123345.

5. Asik, M., Gunes, F., Binnetoglu, E., Eroglu, M., Bozkurt, N., Sen, H., Akbal, E., Bakar, C., Beyazit, Y., Ukinc, K. "Decrease in TSH Levels after Lactose Restriction in Hashimoto's Thyroiditis Patients with Lactose Intolerance." *Endocrine* 46, no. 2 (2014): 279-284. doi: 10.1007/s12020-013-0065-1. PMID: 24078411.

6. Bernareggi, A., Grata, E., Pinorini, M. T., Conti, A. "Oral Liquid Formulation of Levothyroxine is Stable in Breakfast Beverages and May Improve Thyroid Patient Compliance." *Pharmaceutics* 5, no. 4 (2013): 621-633. doi: 10.3390/pharmaceutics5040621. PMID: 24351573; PMCID: PMC3873683.

7. Rees-Jones, R. W., Larsen, P. R. "Triiodothyronine and Thyroxine Content of Desiccated Thyroid Tablets." *Metabolism* 26, no. 11 (1977): 1213-1218. doi: 10.1016/0026-0495(77)90113-5. PMID: 909397.

8. Zhang, Y., Dedkov, E., Teplitsky, D., Weltman, N. Y., Pol, C. J., et al. "Both Hypothyroidism and Hyperthyroidism Increase Atrial Fibrillation Inducibility in Rats." *Circulation: Arrhythmia and Electrophysiology* 6, no. 5 (2013): 952-959.

9. Bauer, M., Fairbanks, L., Berghöfer, A., Hierholzer, J., Bschor, T., Baethge, C., Rasgon, N., Sasse, J., Whybrow, P. C. "Bone Mineral Density During Maintenance Treatment with Supraphysiological Doses of Levothyroxine in Affective Disorders: A Longitudinal Study." *Journal of Affective Disorders* 83, no. 2-3 (2004): 183-190. doi: 10.1016/j.jad.2004.08.011. PMID: 15555712.

10. Watson, C. J., Whitledge, J. D., Siani, A. M., Burns, M. M. "Pharmaceutical Compounding: A History, Regulatory Overview, and Systematic Review of Compounding Errors." *Journal of Medical Toxicology* 17, no. 2 (2021): 197-217. doi: 10.1007/s13181-020-00814-3. Epub 2020 Nov 2. PMID: 33140232; PMCID: PMC7605468.

11. Bolk, N., Visser, T. J., Kalsbeek, A., van Domburg, R. T., Berghout, A. "Effects of Eevening vs Morning Thyroxine Ingestion on Serum Thyroid Hormone Profiles in Hypothyroid Patients." *Clinical Endocrinology (Oxford)* 66, no. 1 (2007): 43-48. doi: 10.1111/j.1365-2265.2006.02681.x. PMID: 17201800.

CHAPTER 10

1. Heini, et al. "Divergent trends in obesity and fat intake patterns: The American Paradox." *American Journal of Medicine* 102, no. 3 (1997): 259-264.

2. Fildes, et al. "Probability of an Obese Person Attaining Normal Body Weight: Cohort Study Using Electronic Health Records." *American Journal of Public Health* 105 (2015): e54_e59.

3. Fothergill, E., Guo, J., Howard, L., Kerns, J. C., Knuth, N. D., Brychta, R., Chen, K. Y., Skarulis, M. C., Walter, M., Walter, P. J., Hall, K. D. "Persistent Metabolic Adaptation 6 Years After *The Biggest Loser* competition." *Obesity (Silver Spring)* 24, no. 8 (2016): 1612-1619. doi: 10.1002/oby.21538. Epub 2016 May 2. PMID: 27136388; PMCID: PMC4989512.

4. Trexler, E. T., Smith-Ryan, A. E., Norton, L. E. "Metabolic Adaptation to Weight Loss: Implications for the Athlete." *Journal of the International Society of Sports Nutrition* 11, no. 1 (2014): 7. doi: 10.1186/1550-2783-11-7. PMID: 24571926; PMCID: PMC3943438.

5. Fung, J. "The Obesity Code." Lulu.com Publishing (2016).

6. "Lipogenesis." *ScienceDirect. URL:* https://www.sciencedirect.com/topics/medicine-and-dentistry/lipogenesis/.

7. Williams, J., Mobarhan, S. "A Critical Interaction: Leptin and Ghrelin." *Nutrition Reviews* 61, no. 11 (2003): 391-393. doi: 10.1301/nr.2003.nov.391-393. PMID: 14677575.

8. Gierach, M., Gierach, J., Junik, R. "Insulin Resistance and Thyroid Disorders." *Endokrynologia Polska* 65, no. 1 (2014): 70-76. doi: 10.5603/EP.2014.0010. PMID: 24549605.

9. Choi, Y. M., Kim, M. K., Kwak, M. K. et al. "Association between Thyroid Hormones and Insulin Resistance Indices Based on the Korean National Health and Nutrition Examination Survey." *Scientific Reports* 11 (2021): 21738.

10. Shapiro, A., Mu, W., Roncal, C., Cheng, K. Y., Johnson, R. J., Scarpace, P. J. "Fructose-Induced Leptin Resistance Exacerbates Weight Gain in Response to Subsequent High-Fat Feeding." *American Journal of Physiology-Regululatory Integrative and Comparative Physiology* 295, no. 5 (2008): R1370-5. doi: 10.1152/ajpregu.00195.2008. Epub 2008 Aug 13. PMID: 18703413; PMCID: PMC2584858.

11. Vibhu Parcha, Brittain Heindl, Rajat Kalra, Peng Li, Barbara Gower, Garima Arora, Pankaj Arora, "Insulin Resistance and Cardiometabolic Risk Profile Among Nondiabetic American Young Adults: Insights From NHANES." *The Journal of Clinical Endocrinology & Metabolism* 107, no. 1 (2022): e25–e37.

12. "Overweight & Obesity Statistics." *National Institute of Diabetes and Digestive and Kidney Diseases. URL:* https://www.niddk.nih. gov/health-information/health-statistics/overweight-obesity/.

CHAPTER 11

1. Hofmekler, O. "The Warrior Diet: Switch on Your Biological Powerhouse for High Energy, Explosive Strength, and a Leaner, Harder Body." Blue Snake Books. (2007).

2. Pilon, B. "Eat Stop Eat: The Shocking Truth That Makes Weight Loss Simple Again." Self-published. (2007).

3. Harrison, K. "The 5:2 Diet: Feast for 5 Days Fast for 2 Days to Lose Weight and Revitalize Your Health." Ulysses Press. (2013).

4. Yuanshan, Tong, et al. "Health Effects of Alternate-Day Fasting in Adults: A Systematic Review and Meta-Analysis." *Frontiers in Nutrition* 7 (2020).

5. "Resources." Toronto Metabolic Clinic Resources. URL: https:// www.torontometabolicclinic.com/resources.html/.

6. Meikle, A. W. "The Interrelationships between Thyroid Dysfunction and Hypogonadism in Men and Boys." *Thyroid* 14, no. 1 Suppl (2004): S17-25. doi: 10.1089/105072504323024552. PMID: 15142373.

7. Dumoulin, S. C., Perret, B. P., Bennet, A. P., Caron, P. J. "Opposite Effects of Thyroid Hormones on Binding Proteins for Steroid Hormones (Sex Hormone-Binding Globulin and Corticosteroid-Binding Globulin) in Humans." *European Journal of Endocrinology* 132, no. 5 (1995): 594-598. doi: 10.1530/eje.0.1320594. Erratum in: *European Journal of Endocrinology* 1995 Sep;133(3):381. PMID: 7749500.

8. Kumar, A., Mohanty, B. P. and Rani, L. "Secretion of Testicular Steroids and Gonadotropins in Hypothyroidism." *Andrologia* 39 (2007): 253-260.

9. Behre, H. M., Simoni, M., Nieschlag, E. "Strong Association between Serum Levels of Leptin and Testosterone in Men." *Clinical Endocrinology (Oxford)* 47, no. 2 (1997): 237-240. doi: 10.1046/j.1365-2265.1997.2681067.x. PMID: 9302400.

10. "High Estrogen: Symptoms, Causes, Diagnosis, and More." Healthline. URL: https://www.healthline.com/health/high-estrogen#diagnosis/.

11. Sathi, P., Kalyan, S., Hitchcock, C. L., Pudek, M., Prior, J. C. "Progesterone Therapy Increases Free Thyroxine Levels—Data from a Randomized Placebo-Controlled 12-Week Hot Fush Trial." *Clinical Endocrinology (Oxford)* 79, no. 2 (2013): 282-287. doi: 10.1111/cen.12128. Epub 2013 May 6. PMID: 23252963.

12. Bertoni, A. P., Brum, I. S., Hillebrand, A. C., Furlanetto, T. W. "Progesterone Upregulates Gene Expression in Normal Human Thyroid Follicular Cells." *International Journal of Endocrinology* (2015): 864852. doi: 10.1155/2015/864852. Epub 2015 May 21. PMID: 26089899; PMCID: PMC4454767.

13. Walter, K. N., Corwin, E. J., Ulbrecht, J., Demers, L. M., Bennett, J. M., Whetzel, C. A., Klein, L. C. "Elevated Thyroid Stimulating Hormone is Associated with Elevated Cortisol in Healthy Young Men and Women." *Thyroid Research* 5, no. 1 (2012): 13. doi: 10.1186/1756-6614-5-13. PMID: 23111240; PMCID: PMC3520819.

14. Samuels, M. H. "Effects of Variations in Physiological Cortisol Levels on Thyrotropin Secretion in Subjects with Adrenal Insufficiency: A Clinical Research Center Study." *The Journal of Clinical Endocrinology & Metabolism* 85, no. 4 (2000): 1388–1393. URL: https://doi.org/10.1210/jcem.85.4.6540

15. Fontana, L., Klein, S., Holloszy, J. O., Premachandra, B. N. "Effect of Long-Term Calorie Restriction with Adequate Protein and Micronutrients on Thyroid Hormones." *The Journal of*

Clinical Endocrinology & Metabolism 91, no. 8 (2006): 3232-3235. doi: 10.1210/jc.2006-0328. Epub 2006 May 23. PMID: 16720655.

16. Spaulding, S. W., Chopra, I. J., Sherwin, R. S., Lyall, S. S. "Effect of Caloric Restriction and Dietary Composition of Serum T3 and Reverse T3 in Man." *The Journal of Clinical Endocrinology & Metabolism* 42, no. 1 (1976): 197-200. doi: 10.1210/jcem-42-1-197. PMID: 1249190.

17. Redman, L. M., Smith, S. R., Burton, J. H., Martin, C. K., Il'yasova, D., Ravussin, E. "Metabolic Slowing and Reduced Oxidative Damage with Sustained Caloric Restriction Support the Rate of Living and Oxidative Damage Theories of Aging." *Cell Metabolism* 27, no. 4 (2018): 805-815.e4. doi: 10.1016/j.cmet.2018.02.019. Epub 2018 Mar 22. PMID: 29576535; PMCID: PMC5886711.

18. Wadden, T. A., Mason, G., Foster, G. D., Stunkard A. J., Prange A. J. "Effects of a Very Low Calorie Diet on Weight, Thyroid Hormones and Mood." *International Journal of Obesity* 14, no. 3 (1990): 249-258. PMID: 2341229.

19. Gearhardt, A. N., Davis, C., Kuschner, R., Brownell, K. D. "The Addiction Potential of Hyperpalatable Foods." *Current Drug Abuse Reviews* 4, no. 3 (2011): 140-145. doi: 10.2174/1874473711104030140. PMID: 21999688.

20. Liu, D., Deng, Y., Sha, L., Abul Hashem M., Gai, S. "Impact of Oral Processing on Texture Attributes and Taste Perception." *Journal of Food Science and Technology* 54, no. 8 (2017): 2585-2593. doi: 10.1007/s13197-017-2661-1. Epub 2017 May 29. PMID: 28740316; PMCID: PMC5502015.

21. Martínez Steele, E., Baraldi, L. G., Louzada, M. L., Moubarac, J. C., Mozaffarian, D., Monteiro, C. A. "Ultra-Processed Foods and Added Sugars in the US Diet: Evidence from a Nationally Representative Cross-Sectional Study." *BMJ Open* 6, no. 3 (2016): e009892. doi: 10.1136/bmjopen-2015-009892. PMID: 26962035; PMCID: PMC4785287.

22. Khobragade, Rahul & Wakode, Santosh. (2018). "Effect of Fasting and Satiety on Taste Perception among Healthy Male Adults." *World Journal of Pharmaceutical and Medical Research* 4, no. 3 (2018): 252-255.

23. "How to Cook Eggs: Scrambled Eggs, Boiled Eggs & More," Jones Dairy Farm. URL: https://www.jonesdairyfarm.com/brinner/how-tos/cook-eggs/.

24. Cava, E., Yeat, N. C., Mittendorfer, B. "Preserving Healthy Muscle during Weight Loss." *Advances in Nutrition* 8, no. 3 (2017): 511-519. doi: 10.3945/an.116.014506. PMID: 28507015; PMCID: PMC5421125.

25. Speed, C. "Exercise and Menstrual Function." *BMJ* 334, no. 7586 (2007): 164-165. doi: 10.1136/bmj.39043.625498.80. PMID: 17255569; PMCID: PMC1781987.

26. Rawal, S. B., Singh, M. V., Tyagi, A. K., Selvamurthy, W., Chaudhuri, B. N. "Effect of Yogic Exercises on Thyroid Function in Subjects Resident at Sea Level upon Exposure to High Altitude." *International Journal of Biometeorology* 38, no. 1 (1994): 44-47. doi: 10.1007/BF01241804. PMID: 8039950.

27. Durmus, D., Alayli, G., Aliyazicioglu, Y., Buyukakıncak, O., Canturk, F. "Effects of Glucosamine Sulfate and Exercise Therapy on Serum Leptin Levels in Patients with Knee Osteoarthritis: Preliminary Results of Randomized Controlled Clinical Trial." *Rheumatology International* 33, no. 3 (2013): 593-599. doi: 10.1007/s00296-012-2401-9. Epub 2012 Apr 3. PMID: 22476244.

28. Marreiro, D. N., Geloneze, B., Tambascia, M. A., Lerário, A. C., Halpern, A., Cozzolino, S. M. "Effect of Zinc Supplementation on Serum Leptin Levels and Insulin Resistance of Obese Women." *Biological Trace Element Research* 112, no. 2 (2006): 109-118. doi: 10.1385/bter:112:2:109. PMID: 17028377.

29. Nelson, F. R., Zvirbulis, R. A., Zonca, B., Li, K. W., Turner, S. M., Pasierb, M., Wilton, P., Martinez-Puig, D., Wu, W. "The Effects of an Oral Preparation Containing Hyaluronic Acid (Oralvisc®) on Obese Knee Osteoarthritis Patients Determined by Pain, Function, Bradykinin, Leptin, Inflammatory Cytokines, and Heavy Water Analyses." *Rheumatology International* 35, no. 1 (2015): 43-52. doi: 10.1007/s00296-014-3047-6. Epub 2014 Jun 5. Erratum in: Rheumatol Int. 2015 Jan;35(1):53. PMID: 24899570.

30. Li, X. X., Li, C. B., Xiao, J., Gao, H. Q., Wang, H. W., Zhang, X. Y., Zhang, C., Ji, X. P. "Berberine Attenuates Vascular Remodeling and Inflammation in a Rat Model of Metabolic Syndrome." *Biological and Pharmaceutical Bulletin* 38, no. 6 (2015): 862-868. doi: 10.1248/bpb.b14-00828. PMID: 26027825.

31. Havel, PJ. "A Scientific Review: The Role of Chromium in Insulin Resistance." *Diabetes Educator* Suppl (2004): 2-14. PMID: 15208835.

32. Lee, W. J., Song, K. H., Koh, E. H., Won, J. C., Kim, H. S., Park, H. S., Kim, M. S., Kim, S. W., Lee, K. U., Park, J. Y. "Alpha-Lipoic Acid Increases Insulin Sensitivity by Activating AMPK in Skeletal Muscle." *Biochemical and Biophysical Research Communications* 332, no. 3 (2005): 885-891. doi: 10.1016/j.bbrc.2005.05.035. PMID: 15913551.

33. DiNicolantonio, J. J. "H O'Keefe JMyo-Inositol for Insulin Resistance, Metabolic Syndrome, Polycystic Ovary Syndrome and Gestational Diabetes." *Open Heart* 9 (2022): e001989. doi: 10.1136/openhrt-2022-001989.

34. Leal-Cerro, A., Soto, A., Martínez, M. A., Dieguez, C., Casanueva, F. F. "Influence of Cortisol Status on Leptin Secretion." *Pituitary* 4, no. 1-2 (2001): 111-116. doi: 10.1023/a:1012903330944. PMID: 11824503.

35. Kingsley, M. "Effects of Phosphatidylserine Supplementation on Exercising Humans. *Sports Medicine* 36, no. 8 (2006): 657-669. doi: 10.2165/00007256-200636080-00003. PMID: 16869708.

36. Panossian, A., Hambardzumyan, M., Hovhanissyan, A., Wikman, G. "The Adaptogens Rhodiola and Schizandra Modify the Response to Immobilization Stress in Rabbits by Suppressing the Increase of Phosphorylated Stress-Activated Protein Kinase, Nitric Oxide and Cortisol." *Drug Target Insights* 2 (2007): 39-54. Epub 2007 Feb 16. PMID: 21901061; PMCID: PMC3155223.

37. Beccuti, G., Pannain, S. "Sleep and Obesity." *Current Opinion in Clinical Nutrition and Metabolic Care* 14, no. 4 (2011): 402-412. doi: 10.1097/MCO.0b013e3283479109. PMID: 21659802; PMCID: PMC3632337.

38. Knutson, K. L., Spiegel, K., Penev, P., Van Cauter, E. "The Metabolic Consequences of Sleep Deprivation." *Sleep Medicine Reviews* 11, no. 3 (2007): 163-178. doi: 10.1016/j. smrv.2007.01.002. Epub 2007 Apr 17. PMID: 17442599; PMCID: PMC1991337.

39. Kanoski S. E., Ong Z. Y., Fortin S. M., Schlessinger E. S., Grill H. J. "Liraglutide, Leptin and their Combined Effects on Feeding: Additive Intake Reduction through Common Intracellular Signaling Mechanisms." *Diabetes Obesity & Metabolism* 17, no. 3 (2015): 285-293. doi: 10.1111/dom.12423. Epub 2015 Jan 8. PMID: 25475828; PMCID: PMC4320650.

40. Lepsen, E. W., Lundgren, J., Dirksen, C., Jensen, J. E., Pedersen, O., Hansen, T., Madsbad, S., Holst, J. J., Torekov, S. S. "Treatment with a GLP-1 Receptor Agonist Diminishes the Decrease in Free Plasma Leptin During Maintenance of Weight Loss." *International Journal of Obesity (London)* 39, no. 5 (2015): 834-841. doi: 10.1038/ijo.2014.177. Epub 2014 Oct 7. PMID: 25287751; PMCID: PMC4424381.

41. Podhorecka, M., Ibanez, B., Dmoszyńska, A. "Metformin - Its Potential Anti-Cancer and Anti-Aging Effects." *Postepy Higieny i Medycyny Doswiadczalnej* (Online) 71, no. 0 (2017): 170-175. doi: 10.5604/01.3001.0010.3801. PMID: 28258677.

42. Baruah, M. P., Kalra, S., Ranabir, S. "Metformin: A character Actor in the Leptin Story!" *Indian Journal of Endocrinology and Metabolism* 16, no. 3 Suppl (2012): S532-533. doi: 10.4103/2230-8210.105569. PMID: 23565486; PMCID: PMC3602980.

43. Yong-Woon Kim, Jong-Yeon Kim, Yong-Hoon Park, So-Young Park, Kyu-Chang Won, Kwang-Hae Choi, Jung-Yoon Huh, Ki-Hak Moon "Metformin Restores Leptin Sensitivity in High-Fat–Fed Obese Rats with Leptin Resistance." *Diabetes* 55, no. 3 (2006): 716–724.

44. Seifarth, C., Schehler, B., Schneider, H. J. "Effectiveness of Metformin on Weight Loss in Non-Diabetic Individuals with Obesity." *Experimental and Clinical Endocrinology & Diabetes* 121, no. 1 (2013): 27-31. doi: 10.1055/s-0032-1327734. Epub 2012 Nov 12. PMID: 23147210.

45. Bihari B. "Bernard Bihari, MD: Low-Dose Naltrexone for Normalizing Immune System Function." *Alternative Therapies in Health and Medicine* 19, no. 2 (2013): 56-65. PMID: 23594453.

46. Kurbanov, D. B., Currie, P. J., Simonson, D. C., Borsook, D., Elman, I. "Effects of Naltrexone on Food Intake and Body Weight Gain in Olanzapine-Treated Rats." *Journal of Psychopharmacology* 26, no. 9 (2012): 1244-1251. doi: 10.1177/0269881112450783. Epub 2012 Jun 21. PMID: 22723540.

47. Xu, L., Ota, T. "Emerging Roles of SGLT2 Inhibitors in Obesity and Insulin Resistance: Focus on Fat Browning and Macrophage Polarization." *Adipocyte* 7, no. 2 (2018): 121-128. doi: 10.1080/21623945.2017.1413516. Epub 2018 Jan 29. PMID: 29376471; PMCID: PMC6152529.

48. Pinto, L. C., Rados, D. V., Remonti, L. R., Kramer, C. K., Leitao, C. B., Gross, J. L. "Efficacy of SGLT2 Inhibitors in Glycemic Control, Weight Loss and Blood Pressure Reduction: A Systematic Review and Meta-Analysis." *Diabetology & Metabolic Syndrome* 7, no. 1 Suppl (2015): A58. doi: 10.1186/1758-5996-7-S1-A58. PMCID: PMC4653505.

49. Eiden, S., Daniel, C., Steinbrueck, A., Schmidt, I., Simon, E. "Salmon Calcitonin - A Potent Inhibitor of Food Intake in States of Impaired Leptin Signaling in Laboratory Rodents." *Journal of Physiology*. 2002 Jun 15;541, no. 3 (2002): 1041-1048. doi: 10.1113/jphysiol.2002.018671. PMID: 12068061; PMCID: PMC2290353.

50. Niall, H. D., Keutmann, H. T., Copp, D. H., Potts, J. T., Jr. "Amino Acid Sequence of Salmon Ultimobranchial Calcitonin." *Proceedings of the National Academy of Sciences of the United States of America* 64, no. 2 (1969): 771-778. doi: 10.1073/pnas.64.2.771. PMID: 5261048; PMCID: PMC223410.

51. Wells, G., Chernoff, J., Gilligan, J. P., Krause, D. S. "Does Salmon Calcitonin Cause Cancer? A Review and Meta-Analysis." *Osteoporosis International* 27, no. 1 (2016): 13-19. doi: 10.1007/s00198-015-3339-z. Epub 2015 Oct 5. PMID: 26438308; PMCID: PMC4715844.

52. De Pergola, G., Silvestris, F. "Obesity as a Major Risk Factor for Cancer." *Journal of Obesity* 2013 (2013): 291546. doi: 10.1155/2013/291546. Epub 2013 Aug 29. PMID: 24073332; PMCID: PMC3773450.

53. "How to Cook Eggs: Scrambled Eggs, Boiled Eggs & More." Jones Dairy Farm. URL: https://www.bodybuildingmealplan.com/reverse-dieting.

54. De Jonge, L., Trump, G. "Does slow reintroduction of calories after weight loss prevent weight regain in trained athletes? A feasibility study." (2017)

55. Darbre, P. D. "Endocrine Disruptors and Obesity." *Current Obesisty Reports* 6, no. 1 (2017): 18-27. doi: 10.1007/s13679-017-0240-4. PMID: 28205155; PMCID: PMC5359373.

56. Kim, K. Y., Lee, E., Kim, Y. "The Association between Bisphenol A Exposure and Obesity in Children-A Systematic Review with Meta-Analysis." *International Journal of Environmental Research and Public Health* 16, no. 14 (2019): 2521. doi: 10.3390/ijerph16142521. PMID: 31311074; PMCID: PMC6678763.

57. Kataria, A., Levine, D., Wertenteil, S. et al. "Exposure to Bisphenols and Phthalates and Association with Oxidant Stress, Insulin Resistance, and Endothelial Dysfunction in Children." *Pediatric Research* 81 (2017): 857–864.

58. Li-Li Wen, Lian-Yu Lin, Ta-Chen Su, Pau-Chung Chen, Chien-Yu Lin, "Association Between Serum Perfluorinated Chemicals and Thyroid Function in U.S. Adults: The National Health and Nutrition Examination Survey 2007–2010," *The Journal of Clinical Endocrinology & Metabolism* 98, no. 9, (2013): E1456–E1464.

59. Shapiro, A., Mu, W., Roncal, C., Cheng, K. Y., Johnson, R. J., Scarpace, P. J. "Fructose-Induced Leptin Resistance Exacerbates Weight Gain in Response to Subsequent High-Fat Feeding." *American Journal of Physiology-Regulatory, Integrative and Comparative Physiology* 295, no. 5 (2008): R1370-1375. doi: 10.1152/ajpregu.00195.2008. Epub 2008 Aug 13. PMID: 18703413; PMCID: PMC2584858.

60. Xiaoli Guo, Qiaoyun Yang, Wei Zhang, Yujiao Chen, Jing Ren, Ai Gao, "Associations of Blood Levels of Trace Elements and Heavy Metals with Metabolic Syndrome in Chinese Male Adults with microRNA as Mediators Involved." *Environmental Pollution* 248 (2019): 66-73. ISSN 0269-7491.

61. Rice, K. M., Walker, E. M., Jr, Wu, M., Gillette, C., Blough, E. R. "Environmental Mercury and its Toxic Effects." *Journal of Preventive Medicine and Public Health* 47, no. 2 (2014): 74-83. doi: 10.3961/jpmph.2014.47.2.74. Epub 2014 Mar31. PMID: 24744824; PMCID: PMC3988285.

CHAPTER 12

1. National Library of Medicine. URL: https://www.ncbi.nlm.nih.gov/pmc/articles/PMC5422478/.

2. National Library of Medicine. URL: https://pubmed.ncbi.nlm.nih.gov/23377335/.

CHAPTER 13

1. "A Patient's Guide to the Diagnosis and Treatment of Hypothyroidism." Thyroid UK. URL: https://thyroiduk.org/further-reading/a-patients-guide-to-the-diagnosis-and-treatment-of-hypothyroidism/.

ABOUT ME

I was raised on a farm in Claude, Texas, with a farmer/coach father and a mother who worked as a custodian at the local nursing home. I attended college at Wayland Baptist University in Plainview, Texas. I then graduated from Texas A&M medical school in 1994 and attended a well-respected family medicine residency program from 1994-1997.

When I began my medical practice in Amarillo, Texas, in 1997, I was excited. I was well-prepared for the busy, complex job of being a physician. The moniker "jack of all trades, master of none" is a great description for a family doctor.

We are taught a little bit of almost every field of medicine, but we don't overly focus on any one field in particular.

Some parts of medicine were still very difficult for me. The area where I felt the most frustration was hormones.

The way I was taught to manage them didn't seem to help them very much.

- My hypothyroid patients still gained weight and felt exhausted even after I started them on levothyroxine.
- I continually saw women in their 40s and 50s who looked and acted like they had major hormone issues. They had irregular periods, libido issues, mood changes, hot flashes, night sweats, and a host of other complaints. All their lab testing was "normal," so there wasn't much to offer them except for meds such as antidepressants, birth control pills or sleep aids.
- My diabetic patients continued to show worsening evidence of organ damage from the disease even though their blood sugars were under pretty good control.
- Middle-aged men were tired, losing their sex drive, losing their muscle mass, and generally felt terrible. Their testosterone levels were in the normal range, so there wasn't much that I knew to offer them.

What was I missing? I knew there must be more that I could be doing, but I didn't know what.

My personal health journey took a major hit in the early 2000s when I contracted a giardia infection in my intestines (I still don't know how or why). It took several rounds of antibiotics to get the infection eradicated (or what I thought was eradicated). My life changed permanently after that. I had constant abdominal cramps with 20 or more diarrhea episodes per day. I slept an average of 4-5 hours per night, because my trips to the bathroom continued throughout the night. I gained over 30 pounds because the only foods that didn't upset my stomach were simple carbs. If I ate a little bit almost constantly, it seemed to settle my stomach.

At the urging of a friend, I finally saw an integrative doctor in another city. I stepped into his office expecting voodoo dolls and crystals, based on my perception of the integrative medicine world. What I found instead was a common sense, personable doctor and staff who were willing to spend a lot of time with me. They changed my diet, gave me some supplements, and explained my situation to me. Within a month, I was 50% better; within 3 months, I was 90% better.

I was bewildered. If integrative medicine had made such a difference with my gut health, what about all the other areas of medicine? What about hormones?

I started reading anything I could find from integrative or functional providers. I read books and blog articles and listened to podcasts from Mark Hyman, Amy Myers, Chris Kresser, Westin Childs, Izabella Wentz, and many others. I attended multiple conferences. I hounded the integrative doctor that helped repair my gut with hundreds of text questions. It was like I was learning medicine all over again (which I was). It all finally started to make sense.

I took a Biote training course and began offering testosterone and estrogen pellet therapy to patients. I saw their worlds change for the better. I was finally doing something that noticeably helped people!

When you start believing and practicing medicine in a way that is not typical, it can become a lonely place. Over the years, my style of practice has cost me some friendships in the medical field. I suppose it just makes many conventional doctors uncomfortable to see things treated in a different way than what they know and were taught. That makes me terribly sad. My critique is not against them; it is against the medical establishment and how slow it is to embrace new and better treatments.

I have been married to my beautiful wife, Pam, for over 34 years. We have three incredible adult children and three (so far) grandchildren.

I feel a passion for helping people who are struggling with thyroid issues. My hope is to get this book in front of whoever needs it so they can start their journey back to health. I also hope that a few medical providers will read it with an open mind. I know it works! Help me get out the message!

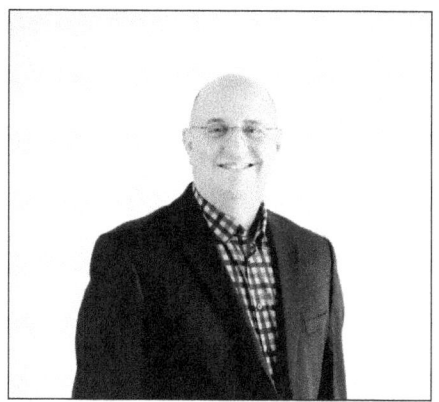

Jeffery Whelchel, MD is the founder and owner of Healthy Hormones PLLC in Amarillo, Texas. He has been in medical practice in Amarillo since 1997. Since 2021, he has focused solely on hormone optimization, especially thyroid and testosterone management. He has been married to his wife Pam since 1989. They have 3 grown children and 3 incredible grandchildren.

www.healthyhormones.us

Dr. Whelchel is available for select lectures, podcasts, or other speaking engagements.

To inquire, please contact him at drjeffhormones@gmail.com or 806-676-5545.